Updates in Clinical Dermatology

Updates in Clinical Dermatology aims to promote the rapid and efficient transfer of medical research into clinical practice. It is published in four volumes per year. Covering new developments and innovations in all fields of clinical dermatology, it provides the clinician with a review and summary of recent research and its implications for clinical practice. Each volume is focused on a clinically relevant topic and explains how research results impact diagnostics, treatment options and procedures as well as patient management. The reader-friendly volumes are highly structured with core messages, summaries, tables, diagrams and illustrations and are written by internationally well-known experts in the field. A volume editor supervises the authors in his/her field of expertise in order to ensure that each volume provides cutting-edge information most relevant and useful for clinical dermatologists. Contributions to the series are peer reviewed by an editorial board.

More information about this series at https://link.springer.com/bookseries/13203

Nicholas Brownstone • Tina Bhutani
Wilson Liao
Editors

Biologic Therapy for Psoriasis

Cutting Edge Treatment Principles

Springer

Editors
Nicholas Brownstone
Psoriasis and Skin Treatment Center
University of California, San Francisco
San Francisco, CA, USA

Tina Bhutani
Psoriasis and Skin Treatment Center
University of California, San Francisco
San Francisco, CA, USA

Wilson Liao
Psoriasis and Skin Treatment Center
University of California, San Francisco
San Francisco, CA, USA

ISSN 2523-8884 ISSN 2523-8892 (electronic)
Updates in Clinical Dermatology
ISBN 978-3-030-92937-4 ISBN 978-3-030-92938-1 (eBook)
https://doi.org/10.1007/978-3-030-92938-1

This Springer imprint is published by the registered company Springer Nature Switzerland AG
The registered company address is: Gewerbestrasse 11, 6330 Cham, Switzerland

NB – I dedicate this book to my parents, Judy and Doug, and my sisters, Nina and Julie

TB – To my children, Kiaan and Haley, and my husband, Glen, for their never-ending support!

Foreword

I am honored to have been asked to write the foreword for this book. Biologic therapy has revolutionized treatment for psoriasis. Moreover, this transformation occurred in an amazingly short time period, well within my career in dermatology. When I started as the Director of the University of California, San Francisco (UCSF) Psoriasis and Skin Treatment Center back in 1988, the main options available for generalized psoriasis were methotrexate, PUVA, and Goeckerman therapy. Cyclosporine was only being tested for FDA approval and most dermatologists stayed away from any internal medications out of fear for possible side effects. This resulted in rampant undertreatment of psoriasis with consequently untold misery for the patients. Today, biologics have spearheaded the transformation of our specialty, where systemic agents are much more widely accepted by dermatologists. Along with all the providers in dermatology, I am fortunate to have witnessed this incredible transformation; I truly feel like Orville Wright (of the Wright Brothers) who became the first human being to fly on an airplane and live to see its evolution into jet planes.

This book is the most up to date and clinically useful source of information for biologic treatments of psoriasis. In this critically important area of dermatological day-to-day practice, any busy clinician or trainee in dermatology will find this book indispensable. Moreover, this book is written with such clarity and user friendliness that it will not only teach you highly relevant practical tips, but it will also be enjoyable to read. I am certain this book will enhance your knowledge which will help patients with all different types of psoriatic disease who are treated with biologic therapy.

San Francisco, CA, USA John Koo

Preface

As is true with the practice of medicine, the treatment of psoriasis with biologic agents is both an art and a science. Given that there are now over 10 FDA-approved biologic agents for psoriasis (with more in the pipeline), confusion exists among providers regarding which agent is best for a particular patient. This book will cover all FDA-approved biologic agents as well as pipeline agents for use in pediatric and adult patients. This book is unique in that it will not only cover cutting-edge treatment principles based on the latest research but will also be one of the most comprehensive reviews of psoriasis biologics in the COVID-19 era. Highlights of this book include discussions on treatment of special sites (genital, scalp, and nail disease), treatment in special populations (e.g., elderly, patients with a history of malignancy, and those undergoing surgery), and how to optimize patient compliance with biologic therapy. We believe that practicing dermatologists and rheumatologists, dermatology and rheumatology trainees, and medical students will all have something new to learn from this book.

The authors contributing to this book have outstanding expertise in the field of psoriasis and biologic therapy. Because general treatment principles do not change, even as novel agents are released, we expect this book to be relevant for many years. The ultimate goal of this book is to improve patient care by making the busy practitioner more adept and comfortable with the use of these particular therapies. If the knowledge you gain from reading this book helps even one patient, we view that as a success!

San Francisco, CA, USA — Nicholas Brownstone
San Francisco, CA, USA — Tina Bhutani
San Francisco, CA, USA — Wilson Liao

Acknowledgements

The editors would like to thank Howard Maibach, MD and the entire clinical and administrative staff of the UCSF Psoriasis and Skin Treatment Center.

Contents

Contributors

Esther A. Balogh, MD Center for Dermatology Research, Department of Dermatology, Wake Forest School of Medicine, Winston-Salem, NC, USA

Tina Bhutani, MD, MAS Department of Dermatology, Psoriasis and Skin Treatment Center, University of California, San Francisco, San Francisco, CA, USA

Nicholas Brownstone, MD Department of Dermatology, Psoriasis and Skin Treatment Center, University of California, San Francisco, San Francisco, CA, USA

Kelly M. Cordoro, MD University of California San Francisco, Department of Dermatology, San Francisco, CA, USA

Deborah Cull, BSE Center for Dermatology Research, Department of Dermatology, Wake Forest School of Medicine, Winston-Salem, NC, USA

Steven R. Feldman, MD, PhD Center for Dermatology Research, Department of Dermatology, Wake Forest School of Medicine, Winston-Salem, NC, USA

Department of Pathology, Wake Forest School of Medicine, Winston-Salem, NC, USA

Department of Social Sciences & Health Policy, Wake Forest School of Medicine, Winston-Salem, NC, USA

Department of Dermatology, University of Southern Denmark, Odense, Denmark

Center for Dermatology Research, Wake Forest School of Medicine, Winston-Salem, NC, USA

Edward Hadeler, BA University of California, San Francisco, Department of Dermatology, Psoriasis and Skin Treatment Center, San Francisco, CA, USA

University of Miami Leonard M. Miller School of Medicine, Miami, FL, USA

Marwa Hakimi, MD University of California, San Francisco, Department of Dermatology, Psoriasis and Skin Treatment Center, San Francisco, CA, USA

George Han, MD, PhD Icahn School of Medicine at Mount Sinai, New York City, NY, USA

Jason E. Hawkes, MD, MS Department of Dermatology, University of California-Davis, Sacramento, CA, USA

Julie Hong, BS University of California, San Francisco, Department of Dermatology, Psoriasis and Skin Treatment Center, San Francisco, CA, USA

Pennsylvania State University College of Medicine, Hershey, PA, USA

Momoko Ishizuka, BS Southern California Dermatology, Inc., Santa Ana, CA, USA

Harbor University of California, Los Angeles, CA, USA

John Koo, MD Department of Dermatology, Psoriasis and Skin Treatment Center, University of California, San Francisco, San Francisco, CA, USA

Mark Lebwohl, MD Department of Dermatology, Icahn School of Medicine at Mount Sinai Hospital, New York, NY, USA

Wilson Liao, MD University of California, San Francisco, Department of Dermatology, Psoriasis and Skin Treatment Center, San Francisco, CA, USA

Jeffrey Liu, BS Keck School of Medicine, University of Southern California, Los Angeles, CA, USA

Alexandra Mari, DO Eastern Virginia Medical School Department of Infectious Disease/Critical Care, Norfolk, VA, USA

Amylee Martin, BS School of Medicine, University of California, Riverside, CA, USA

Megan Mosca, BS University of California, San Francisco, Department of Dermatology, Psoriasis and Skin Treatment Center, San Francisco, CA, USA

University of Nevada, Reno School of Medicine, Reno, NV, USA

Mio Nakamura, MD, MS Department of Dermatology, University of Michigan, Ann Arbor, MI, USA

Katie A. O'Connell, MS Eastern Virginia Medical School Department of Dermatology, Norfolk, VA, USA

Joseph Pena, MS Center for Dermatology Research, Department of Dermatology, Wake Forest School of Medicine, Winston-Salem, NC, USA

Patrick O. Perche, BS Center for Dermatology Research, Wake Forest School of Medicine, Winston-Salem, NC, USA

Kourtney Pony, BS University of Michigan Medical School, Ann Arbor, MI, USA

Caitlin G. Purvis, BS Center for Dermatology Research, Department of Dermatology, Wake Forest School of Medicine, Winston-Salem, NC, USA

Varun K. Ranpariya, BA Center for Dermatology Research, Wake Forest School of Medicine, Winston-Salem, NC, USA

Jennifer Soung, MD Southern California Dermatology, Inc., Santa Ana, CA, USA

Harbor University of California, Los Angeles, CA, USA

Samuel Stetkevich, BS Southern California Dermatology, Inc., Santa Ana, CA, USA

Harbor University of California, Los Angeles, CA, USA

Qisi Sun, MD Department of Dermatology, Yale University School of Medicine, New Haven, CT, USA

Akshitha Thatiparthi, BS College of Osteopathic Medicine of the Pacific, Western University of Health Sciences, Pomona, CA, USA

Abby S. Van Voorhees, MD Eastern Virginia Medical School Department of Dermatology, Norfolk, VA, USA

Mark Weingarten, BA Icahn School of Medicine at Mount Sinai Hospital, New York, NY, USA

Jashin J. Wu, MD Dermatology Research and Education Foundation, Irvine, CA, USA

Introduction to Biologic Therapy for Psoriasis

1

Nicholas Brownstone and John Koo

What Is Psoriasis?

Psoriasis is an immune-mediated inflammatory skin disease characterized by discrete, erythematous plaques and papules with micaceous scale (Fig. 1.1) [1]. This common disease affects more than 125 million people worldwide [2]. It can present at any age and has been reported at birth and in older individuals as well. The mean age of onset can range from 15 to 20 years of age with a second peak occurring at 55 to 60 years of age [3]. Psoriasis commonly affects the following body areas: knees, elbows, lumbosacral region, scalp, and genital area. However, any area of the body can be affected by psoriasis. From a clinical perspective, psoriasis can present in various forms. Some of these forms include plaque psoriasis, guttate psoriasis, erythrodermic psoriasis, palmoplantar psoriasis, inverse psoriasis, and generalized pustular psoriasis [4]. Psoriasis can also cause nail dystrophy that can sometimes be mistaken for onychomycosis. A unique feature of psoriasis is that it may also develop at the site of trauma or injury, known as Koebner's phenomenon [5].

Psoriasis does not only affect the skin. Evidence shows an association with inflammatory arthritis (psoriatic arthritis), depression, inflammatory bowel disease, metabolic syndrome, and cardiovascular disease [6]. Psoriatic arthritis is a heterogenous, usually seronegative, chronic inflammatory joint disease that is characterized by edema, pain, and stiffness of joints, ligaments, and tendons [7]. Psoriasis patients have a 2.9 times higher risk of developing inflammatory bowel disease compared with the general population [8]. Among the biologic agents that are used to treat psoriasis, some are also used to treat psoriatic arthritis and inflam-

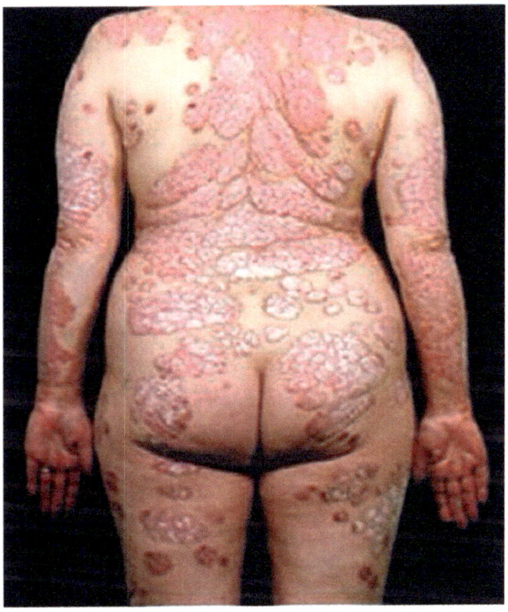

Fig. 1.1 Psoriasis vulgaris

N. Brownstone (✉) · J. Koo
Department of Dermatology, Psoriasis and Skin Treatment Center, University of California, San Francisco, San Francisco, CA, USA

N. Brownstone et al. (eds.), *Biologic Therapy for Psoriasis*, Updates in Clinical Dermatology,
https://doi.org/10.1007/978-3-030-92938-1_1

matory bowel disease. There is a higher incidence of cardiovascular events in psoriasis patients, and psoriasis is thought to provide an additional and independent cardiovascular risk factor given that it is a chronic inflammatory disorder [9]. For example, myocardial infarction (MI) events in patients with psoriasis occur on average 5 years earlier in life than in those patients with MI without psoriasis [10]. Despite this higher risk, Wu et al. demonstrated that the use of biologic agents for psoriasis (TNF-alpha inhibitors) was associated with a significant reduction in MI risk and incident rate compared with topical treatment [11].

Besides physical comorbidities, psoriasis has a marked effect on mental health and quality of life. About 10% of patients with psoriasis have previously considered the possibility of suicide [12]. Surprisingly, the physical, emotional, and social impact of psoriasis on quality of life is similar and sometimes even worse than that observed in patients with major medical conditions such as ischemic heart disease, cancer, arthritis, and diabetes mellitus [13]. Biologic therapy can improve depressive symptoms. One study revealed that patients with psoriasis who were treated with etanercept (a TNF-alpha inhibitor) showed significant decrease in severity/frequency of depressive episodes which correlated with improving skin lesions [14]. Another study by Bhutani et al. demonstrated that based on the Psychological General-Well Being (PGWB) index, patients who were treated with adalimumab began to show improvement in their quality of life by week 4, and by week 24, all six PGWB domains showed statistically significant improvement from pre-treatment baseline [15]. This study also revealed that patients with untreated psoriasis had as much psychological impairment in their well-being as patients with other major medical disorders such as breast cancer, coronary artery disease, congestive heart failure, and diabetes; treatment with adalimumab improved psychological well-being to where it was comparable to patients with asymptomatic hypertension.

Pathophysiology of Psoriasis

Decades of research into the pathophysiology of psoriasis has highlighted the importance of the immune system in the pathophysiology of this disease. A variety of cell types are involved which include keratinocytes, natural killer T cells, plasmacytoid dendritic cells, and macrophages. These cells secrete cytokines which activate myeloid dendritic cells, and in turn, activated myeloid dendritic cells secrete IL-12 and IL-23. Both of these cytokines are integral in the cellular cascade of psoriasis pathophysiology. IL-12 causes differentiation of native T cells to Th1 cells (which produce IFN-γ and TNF-α), and IL-23 is important for the proliferation of Th17 and Th22 cells. Th17 cells produce IL-17, IL-22, and TNF-α [16]. When considering all of these different molecular signaling pathways, IL-23-mediated activation of the Th17 pathway is hypothesized to be the main contributor to the inflammation seen in psoriasis [17].

The fact that biologic agents interact with a specific cytokine (such as TNF-α, IL-17, or IL-23) in a targeted manner has revolutionized the ability to treat psoriasis compared to the era of a more generalized immunosuppression reflected by the traditional systemic medications such as methotrexate or cyclosporine. This targeted immunomodulation has resulted in a great enhancement in both safety and efficacy for biologic agents.

An Introduction to Biologics and a Review of Non-Biologic Systemic Medications for Psoriasis

Biologics are medications whose active component is derived from a biological source by being produced in microorganisms and cells (humans and animals) using biotechnology [18]. Biologics have revolutionized the care of many diseases and have increased the amount of treatment options for complex diseases such as diabetes, cancer, and autoimmune diseases [19]. Based on their pharmacological action, biologics can generally be categorized into those with regulating activity (e.g., recombinant proteins, cytokines), specific targeting capability (e.g., monoclonal antibodies), vaccines, and diagnostics [20]. Most biologic agents for psoriasis fall under the subcategory of monoclonal antibodies. Monoclonal antibodies (mAbs) are antibodies produced by a single clone of B cells, as opposed to polyclonal antibodies, and are monospecific and homogeneous [21]. In the last two decades, the creation of biologics has revolutionized the management of psoriasis. Over this time period, numerous biologic agents have been approved for the treatment of psoriasis, and more are currently in development [22].

Before the advent of biologic agents for psoriasis, oral systemic medications were used that often were not as effective, had serious side effects, or could not be continued indefinitely. Acitretin is an oral retinoid that is fortunately not an immunosuppressive medication and therefore safe in patients with HIV, hepatitis, or infections. It is one of the treatments of choice in pustular psoriasis. Improvement occurs slowly and it typically takes 3–6 months to reach maximal efficacy [23]. Another unique feature of acitretin in dermatology is its use in chemoprevention of nonmelanoma skin cancer (NMSC). Low-dose acitretin (less than 25 mg/day) carries few side effects, both in the short and long term. One popular way that acitretin can be used is in combination with phototherapy for recalcitrant cases of psoriasis [23]. Acitretin cannot be used during pregnancy and pregnancy is not recommended within 3 years of discontinuation of treatment. Other side effects include hyperlipidemia, hepatotoxicity, myalgias, and arthralgias. Laboratory monitoring is recommended every 3 months [23].

Methotrexate is a drug that has the ability to inhibit cellular proliferation by reducing purine and pyrimidine synthesis. It is well established as a competitive inhibitor of dihydrofolate reductase, and thereby prevents the regeneration from dihydrofolate of tetrahydrofolate, which is essential for the generation of folate cofactors required for de novo purine and pyrimidine synthesis. Methotrexate has been used to successfully treat plaque, guttate, pustular, and erythrodermic forms of psoriasis [24]. Major adverse effects of methotrexate include hepatotoxicity (principally in the form of fibrosis) and bone marrow suppression [25]. Based on numerous studies, it is accurate to state that methotrexate, reasonably dosed and over 4 months of continuous therapy, has a PASI 75 achievement rate of approximately 40% [26]. Pregnancy and lactation is an absolute contraindication. Side effects include the possibility of methotrexate-induced liver fibrosis and pancytopenia. More common side effects are nausea, anorexia, ulcerative stomatitis, and diarrhea [26]. Lab monitoring is recommended every 2–3 months.

Lastly, cyclosporine is another systemic medication that has been used for psoriasis before the advent of biologic therapy. Cyclosporine inhibits T-cell activation by selectively inhibiting calcineurin phosphatase, thus suppressing production of IL-2. It has been FDA approved for the treatment of psoriasis since 1997. Cyclosporine is highly effective in treating psoriasis and has been shown to lead to improvement in 80% of patients when used for a period of 12–16 weeks [27]. Cyclosporine is effective in recalcitrant psoriasis, erythrodermic psoriasis, nail psoriasis, and psoriatic arthritis and is well known to rapidly clear widespread and erythrodermic psoriasis. Side effects include nephrotoxicity, hypertension, hyperlipidemia, and neurotoxicity. Due to these side effects, lab monitoring and physical exam are recommended every 1–2 months [28].

An Overview of Biologic Therapy in Psoriasis

The fact that biologic agents interact with a specific cytokine (such as TNF-α, IL-17, or IL-23) in a targeted manner has revolutionized the capacity to treat psoriasis compared to the era of a more generalized immunosuppression and potentially serious side effects reflected by the traditional oral medications discussed above. This represents an improved treatment regimen where targeted immunomodulation has resulted in a great enhancement in both safety and efficacy for biologic agents. There are now over ten FDA-approved biologic agents for psoriasis, with more in the pipeline. Given the numerous options, the treatment of psoriasis with biologic agents is both an art and a science. Biologic agents for the treatment of psoriasis are classified by which cytokine they block. These include TNF-alpha blockers, interleukin (IL)-17 blockers, IL-12/23 blockers, and IL-23 blockers. Many biologic medications have FDA-approved indications for other diseases besides psoriasis, and many agents have FDA approval for psoriatic arthritis. Each biologic agent has a unique merit and even the older agents are still useful in today's therapeutic landscape.

For example, etanercept which was FDA approved for psoriasis in 2004 may no longer be considered first line because of its limited efficacy. However, it is important to remember that etanercept has one of the best FDA "geriatric statements" attesting to its safety in older patients. The package insert states that the risk for elderly patients is nearly the same as the risk for younger patients. Other biologic agents either state the opposite (i.e., older patients are at greater risk than younger patients, such as adalimumab) or have no geriatric statement because of lack of data in this population.

Another example is certolizumab, which has data in human use for over 20 years and can easily be forgotten with the assumption that it has less efficacy than new medications. In reality, the PASI 75 achievement rate of certolizumab approaches that of the newer IL-17 agents. Moreover, being an anti-TNF biologic, its efficacy for psoriatic arthritis is one of the best, which may not be matched by the newest IL-23 agents. Moreover, being an anti-TNF biologic, it can actually treat inflammatory bowel disease as one of the official FDA indications. Certolizumab also has data which shows that it is safe for use in pregnant and breastfeeding patients [29, 30].

Lastly, some may dismiss tildrakizumab as just another IL-23 agent, with a slower onset of action and no further advantages in clinical efficacy. However, on close examination, tildrakizumab is the only biologic agent guaranteed to be covered by Medicare part B due to the requirement that this medication be administered by the healthcare provider, not self-administered. Moreover, tildrakizumab has the smallest list of adverse events (occurring in at least 1% of subjects) that occurred during the phase III clinical trials. Therefore, clinicians who are interested in safety may find this fact very attractive, especially in elderly Medicare patients. Please refer to Table 1.1 for a complete list of current and pipeline biologic agents for the treatment of psoriasis, along with their dosing regimens.

Psoriasis Outcome Measures

In clinical practice, the assessment of psoriasis is relatively easy. Physicians examine the patient's body to get an overall assessment of severity and also ask the patient how they are doing and if they have improved since their last visit. However, in clinical trials more objective measures are needed to be able to reproduce results between different investigators and to compare agents. These systems are needed because when conducting a clinical trial for the treatment for psoriasis, a predetermined primary and reproducible endpoint is required on which the efficacy of the drug will be assessed [31]. Different scoring systems exist to objectively measure psoriasis severity and total area involved. The traditional gold standard for assessment of extensive psoriasis has been the Psoriasis Area and Severity Index (PASI) [32]. The PASI is a measure of the average erythema, thickness, and scaliness of the lesions (each graded on a 0–4 scale), weighted by the area of involvement in different body sites. For example, psoriasis that is covering the left lower extremity will receive a greater score than psoriasis covering the scalp given that there is more body surface area on the left lower extremity. For patients with severe psoriasis, researchers typically consider at least a 75% improvement in disease to be a clinically meaningful improvement

Table 1.1 Biologic treatments of psoriasis

Medication, year of FDA approval	Brand name	Dosing regimen	Alternative dosing regimen
TNF-alpha inhibitors			
Adalimumab, 2002	Humira®	80 mg SC at week 0, 40 mg at week 1, then 40 mg SC q2w	
Etanercept, 2004	Enbrel®	50 mg SC q twice weekly for the first 12 weeks, then 50 mg SC weekly	
Infliximab, 2006	Remicade®	5 mg/kg IV at weeks 0, 2, and 6 and thereafter every 8 weeks	
Certolizumab pegol, 2008	Cimzia®	Patient weight >90 kg: 400 mg SC q2w	Patient weight <90 kg: 400 mg SC at weeks 0, 2, and 4, then 200 mg SC q2w
IL-17 inhibitors			
Secukinumab, 2015	Cosentyx®	300 mg SC at weeks 0, 1, 2, 3, 4, then 300 mg SC q4w	Low body weight and minimal disease severity: 150 mg maintenance q4w
Brodalumab, 2017	Siliq®	210 mg SC at weeks 0, 1, and 2, then 210 mg SC q2w	
Ixekizumab, 2017	Taltz®	160 mg SC at week 0; 80 mg at weeks 2, 4, 6, 8, 10, 12; then 80 mg SC q4w	Maintain treatment response: 80 mg SC q2w
Bimekizumab	N/A		
IL-23 inhibitors			
Guselkumab, 2017	Tremfya®	100 mg SC at weeks 0 and 4, then 100 mg q8w	
Tildrakizumab, 2018	Ilumya®	100 mg at weeks 0 and 4, then 100 mg SC q12w	
Risankizumab, 2019	Skyrizi®	150 mg SC at weeks 0 and 4, then 150 mg q12w	
Mirikizumab	N/A		
IL-12/23 inhibitor			
Ustekinumab, 2009	Stelara®	Patient weight <100 kg: 45 mg SC at weeks 0 and 4, then 45 mg SC q12w Patient weight >100kg, 90 mg SC at weeks 0 and 4, then 90 mg SC q12w	Pediatric patient weight < 60 kg: weight-based dose of 0.75 mg/kg Patient weight 60–100 kg, 45 mg SC Patient weight >100 kg, 90 mg SC

indicative of success. This has been translated into 75% improvement in the PASI score. This scale is widely known and used in most clinical trials and is accepted by key regulatory agencies. It does have some limitations, one of which is its poor sensitivity to change for relatively small areas of involvement. It also is rarely used in clinical practice to assess psoriasis severity.

Another key measure used in clinical trials of psoriasis is the physician global assessment [33]. This is usually a 5-point scoring system where 0 means clear and 4 means very severe psoriasis. Each number has a specific definition to guide the provider in choosing that score. As with the PASI score, the disadvantage here is that it is difficult to detect small changes and the range is relatively restricted. Other psoriasis measurement tools are being developed such as the lattice system. This provides a global psoriasis score that ranges over eight steps from clear to very severe. The investigator rates the elevation (also termed induration or thickness in other measures), erythema, and scaliness of the lesion, each on a none to mild, moderate, marked scale. The percentage of body surface area involved is also measured [34].

Quality of life can be measured in different ways and is an important part of psoriasis clinical trials and psoriasis research. Nonspecific measures such as the Medical Outcome Survey Short Form 36 (SF-36) and the EuroQoL measures assess patients' overall quality of life [35]. There are more specific instruments that focus on aspects of quality of life that are affected by skin disease. These include the Dermatology Life Quality Index (DLQI) and the Skindex [36]. In summary, there is no one best measure for evaluation of psoriasis severity in clinical trials. The PASI, along with physician global assessment and quality of life measures, provides a complement of measures for studies of psoriasis that offer impartiality, are easily interpreted by clinicians, and yield a comprehensive view of the impact of disease [37]. Many studies will use multiple methods of assessment as secondary endpoints to mitigate the disadvantages that come with each measure.

Conclusion

Psoriasis is a common and immune-mediated inflammatory skin disease. Older systemic medications for psoriasis were effective, but some were considered true immunosuppressants and carried undesirable and sometimes serious side effects. Biologic therapy for psoriasis has revolutionized treatment which resulted from discovering the immune dysregulation that is central to the pathophysiology of psoriasis. While most patients with mild psoriasis are managed effectively with topical corticosteroids, biologic agents are necessary for complex, widespread, erythrodermic, and comorbid psoriatic disease. If the decision to start a biologic agent is not so clear-cut, the Koo-Menter Psoriasis instrument (KMPI) may be used to help identify patients that would benefit from biologic therapy and can even be used to document and justify treatment decisions for healthcare payers [38].

The newer biologic agents are nearly able to clear full body psoriasis and are proving to be a safer option compared to the original oral systemic agents. Given there are now over ten different biologic agents FDA approved for psoriasis (with more in the pipeline), it is recommended to not dismiss any biologic agent on just a cursory glance. The nuanced differences between the unique merits of each agent could prove to be very important in improving patient care and patient satisfaction.

References

1. Raju SS. Psoriasis and lasting implications. Expert Rev Clin Immunol. 2014;10(2):175–7. https://doi.org/10.1586/1744666X.2014.872033.
2. Thatiparthi A, Martin A, Liu J, Egeberg A, Wu JJ. Biologic treatment algorithms for moderate-to-severe psoriasis with comorbid conditions and special populations: a review. Am J Clin Dermatol. 2021;22(4):425–42. https://doi.org/10.1007/s40257-021-00603-w.
3. Ferrándiz C, Pujol RM, García-Patos V, Bordas X, Smandía JA. Psoriasis of early and late onset: a clinical and epidemiologic study from Spain. J Am Acad Dermatol. 2002;46(6):867–73. https://doi.org/10.1067/mjd.2002.120470.

4. Sarac G, Koca TT, Baglan T. A brief summary of clinical types of psoriasis. North Clin Istanb. 2016;3(1):79–82. https://doi.org/10.14744/nci.2016.16023.
5. Langley RGB, Krueger GG, Griffiths CEM. Psoriasis: epidemiology, clinical features, and quality of life. Ann Rheum Dis. 2005;64 Suppl 2:ii18–23; discussion ii24-25. https://doi.org/10.1136/ard.2004.033217.
6. Oliveira M de FSP d, Rocha B de O, Duarte GV. Psoriasis: classical and emerging comorbidities. An Bras Dermatol. 2015;90(1):9–20. https://doi.org/10.1590/abd1806-4841.20153038.
7. Moll JM, Wright V. Psoriatic arthritis. Semin Arthritis Rheum. 1973;3(1):55–78. https://doi.org/10.1016/0049-0172(73)90035-8.
8. Gulliver W. Long-term prognosis in patients with psoriasis. Br J Dermatol. 2008;159 Suppl 2:2–9. https://doi.org/10.1111/j.1365-2133.2008.08779.x.
9. Masson W, Lobo M, Molinero G. Psoriasis and cardiovascular risk: a comprehensive review. Adv Ther. 2020;37(5):2017–33. https://doi.org/10.1007/s12325-020-01346-6.
10. Karbach S, Hobohm L, Wild J, et al. Impact of psoriasis on mortality rate and outcome in myocardial infarction. J Am Heart Assoc. 2020;9(18):e016956. https://doi.org/10.1161/JAHA.120.016956.
11. Wu JJ, Poon K-YT, Channual JC, Shen AY-J. Association between tumor necrosis factor inhibitor therapy and myocardial infarction risk in patients with psoriasis. Arch Dermatol. 2012;148(11):1244. https://doi.org/10.1001/archdermatol.2012.2502.
12. Gupta MA, Gupta AK. Depression and suicidal ideation in dermatology patients with acne, alopecia areata, atopic dermatitis and psoriasis. Br J Dermatol. 1998;139(5):846–50. https://doi.org/10.1046/j.1365-2133.1998.02511.x.
13. Rapp SR, Feldman SR, Exum ML, Fleischer AB, Reboussin DM. Psoriasis causes as much disability as other major medical diseases. J Am Acad Dermatol. 1999;41(3 Pt 1):401–7. https://doi.org/10.1016/s0190-9622(99)70112-x.
14. Tyring S, Gottlieb A, Papp K, et al. Etanercept and clinical outcomes, fatigue, and depression in psoriasis: double-blind placebo-controlled randomised phase III trial. Lancet. 2006;367(9504):29–35. https://doi.org/10.1016/S0140-6736(05)67763-X.
15. Bhutani T, Patel T, Koo B, Nguyen T, Hong J, Koo J. A prospective, interventional assessment of psoriasis quality of life using a nonskin-specific validated instrument that allows comparison with other major medical conditions. J Am Acad Dermatol. 2013;69(2):e79–88. https://doi.org/10.1016/j.jaad.2012.10.009.
16. Armstrong AW, Read C. Pathophysiology, clinical presentation, and treatment of psoriasis: a review. JAMA. 2020;323(19):1945–60. https://doi.org/10.1001/jama.2020.4006.
17. Alwan W, Nestle FO. Pathogenesis and treatment of psoriasis: exploiting pathophysiological pathways for precision medicine. Clin Exp Rheumatol. 2015;33(5 Suppl 93):S2–6.
18. Giezen TJ, Mantel-Teeuwisse AK, Straus SMJM, Schellekens H, Leufkens HGM, Egberts ACG. Safety-related regulatory actions for biologicals approved in the United States and the European Union. JAMA. 2008;300(16):1887–96. https://doi.org/10.1001/jama.300.16.1887.
19. Schellekens H. Recombinant human erythropoietins, biosimilars and immunogenicity. J Nephrol. 2008;21(4):497–502.
20. Leader B, Baca QJ, Golan DE. Protein therapeutics: a summary and pharmacological classification. Nat Rev Drug Discov. 2008;7(1):21–39. https://doi.org/10.1038/nrd2399.
21. Breedveld FC. Therapeutic monoclonal antibodies. Lancet. 2000;355(9205):735–40. https://doi.org/10.1016/s0140-6736(00)01034-5.
22. Kim HJ, Lebwohl MG. Biologics and psoriasis: the beat goes on. Dermatol Clin. 2019;37(1):29–36. https://doi.org/10.1016/j.det.2018.07.004.
23. Lee CS, Li K. A review of acitretin for the treatment of psoriasis. Expert Opin Drug Saf. 2009;8(6):769–79. https://doi.org/10.1517/14740330903393732.
24. Chan ESL, Cronstein BN. Methotrexate – how does it really work? Nat Rev Rheumatol. 2010;6(3):175–8. https://doi.org/10.1038/nrrheum.2010.5.
25. Kremer JM, Galivan J, Streckfuss A, Kamen B. Methotrexate metabolism analysis in blood and liver of rheumatoid arthritis patients. Association with hepatic folate deficiency and formation of polyglutamates. Arthritis Rheum. 1986;29(7):832–5. https://doi.org/10.1002/art.1780290703.
26. Strober BE. Methotrexate and cyclosporine in psoriasis revisited. Semin Cutan Med Surg. 2014;33(2 Suppl 2):S27–30. https://doi.org/10.12788/j.sder.0066.
27. Rosmarin DM, Lebwohl M, Elewski BE, Gottlieb AB, National Psoriasis Foundation. Cyclosporine and psoriasis: 2008 National Psoriasis Foundation Consensus Conference. J Am Acad Dermatol. 2010;62(5):838–53. https://doi.org/10.1016/j.jaad.2009.05.017.
28. Amber T, Tabassum S. Cyclosporin in dermatology: a practical compendium. Dermatol Ther. 2020;33(6):e13934. https://doi.org/10.1111/dth.13934.
29. Clowse ME, Förger F, Hwang C, et al. Minimal to no transfer of certolizumab pegol into breast milk: results from CRADLE, a prospective, postmarketing, multicentre, pharmacokinetic study. Ann Rheum Dis. 2017;76(11):1890–6. https://doi.org/10.1136/annrheumdis-2017-211384.
30. Mariette X, Förger F, Abraham B, et al. Lack of placental transfer of certolizumab pegol during pregnancy: results from CRIB, a prospective, postmarketing, pharmacokinetic study. Ann Rheum Dis. 2018;77(2):228–33. https://doi.org/10.1136/annrheumdis-2017-212196.
31. Feldman SR. The design of clinical trials in psoriasis: lessons for clinical practice. J Am Acad Dermatol.

2003;49(2 Suppl):S62–5. https://doi.org/10.1016/s0190-9622(03)01137-x.
32. Fredriksson T, Pettersson U. Severe psoriasis – oral therapy with a new retinoid. Dermatologica. 1978;157(4):238–44. https://doi.org/10.1159/000250839.
33. Pascoe VL, Enamandram M, Corey KC, et al. Using the Physician Global Assessment in a clinical setting to measure and track patient outcomes. JAMA Dermatol. 2015;151(4):375–81. https://doi.org/10.1001/jamadermatol.2014.3513.
34. Langley RG, Ellis CN. Evaluating psoriasis with psoriasis area and severity index, psoriasis global assessment, and lattice system physician's global assessment. J Am Acad Dermatol. 2004;51(4):563–9. https://doi.org/10.1016/j.jaad.2004.04.012.
35. Anderson RT, Aaronson NK, Wilkin D. Critical review of the international assessments of health-related quality of life. Qual Life Res Int J Qual Life Asp Treat Care Rehabil. 1993;2(6):369–95. https://doi.org/10.1007/BF00422215.
36. Finlay AY, Khan GK. Dermatology Life Quality Index (DLQI) – a simple practical measure for routine clinical use. Clin Exp Dermatol. 1994;19(3):210–6. https://doi.org/10.1111/j.1365-2230.1994.tb01167.x.
37. Feldman SR, Krueger GG. Psoriasis assessment tools in clinical trials. Ann Rheum Dis. 2005;64 Suppl 2:ii65–8; discussion ii69–73. https://doi.org/10.1136/ard.2004.031237.
38. Feldman SR, Koo JYM, Menter A, Bagel J. Decision points for the initiation of systemic treatment for psoriasis. J Am Acad Dermatol. 2005;53(1):101–7. https://doi.org/10.1016/j.jaad.2005.03.050.

2 Laboratory Monitoring: HIV, TB and Hepatitis

Katie A. O'Connell, Alexandra Mari, and Abby S. Van Voorhees

Introduction

Patients with moderate-to-severe plaque psoriasis are often treated with biologic therapy to adequately control disease; however the use of biologic therapy can pose potential risks for patients with concomitant chronic infections including human immunodeficiency virus (HIV), tuberculosis (TB), hepatitis B, and hepatitis C. A number of specialty societies and countries have developed guidelines regarding psoriatic disease treatment with biologics, and the vast majority of these guidelines provide evidence-based recommendations regarding pretreatment testing and laboratory monitoring for HIV, TB, hepatitis B, and hepatitis C [1–10]. Here, we discuss the role of HIV, TB, and viral hepatitis screening for psoriasis patients initiating biologic therapy, in addition to ongoing monitoring recommendations.

K. A. O'Connell · A. S. Van Voorhees (✉)
Eastern Virginia Medical School Department of Dermatology, Norfolk, VA, USA
e-mail: oconnek@evms.edu; vanvooas@evms.edu

A. Mari
Eastern Virginia Medical School Department of Infectious Disease/Critical Care, Norfolk, VA, USA
e-mail: maria@evms.edu

Human Immunodeficiency Virus

HIV is an established, independent risk factor for the development of psoriasis, and the prevalence among HIV patients is estimated to be at least as high as that of the general population [11]. Psoriasis may be the initial presentation of HIV infection [12–14]. The sudden onset of psoriasis in healthy individuals with risk factors should raise suspicion for HIV [14–16]. Populations with an increased risk for acquiring HIV are listed in Table 2.1. A higher frequency of guttate, inverse, and erythrodermic subtypes occurs in individuals infected with HIV, but plaque psoriasis remains most frequent in persons living with HIV in western countries [11, 12]. Coexistence of multiple subtypes may also occur more commonly in patients with both psoriasis and HIV. In general, psoriasis becomes more severe with HIV progression and lower CD4 counts. Individuals with a CD4 count <200 are estimated to be nine times more likely to develop psoriasis compared to those with CD4 counts >200 [17]. This paradoxical effect of HIV is well recognized and coincides with more advanced HIV-induced immunosuppression [12].

In patients with preexisting psoriasis, a sudden change in disease pattern or development of refractory disease should prompt a discussion regarding HIV testing [11]. If HIV testing is positive, then it is important to refer the patient to an HIV specialist to begin antiretroviral therapy

N. Brownstone et al. (eds.), *Biologic Therapy for Psoriasis*, Updates in Clinical Dermatology,
https://doi.org/10.1007/978-3-030-92938-1_2

Table 2.1 Risk factors for acquiring disease [2]

Human immunodeficiency virus [18]	Hepatitis B	Hepatitis C [19]	Tuberculosis [20]
IVDA or hx of IVDA MSM ≥1 new sex partner w/ unknown HIV status Sex partner with HIV Commercial sex workers Living in correctional facility or homeless shelter Intranasal cocaine users Recent tattoo Received blood products abroad	IVDA or hx of IVDA MSM History of unprotected sex Multiple sexual partners History of STI Commercial sex workers Living in correctional facility Born or brought up in country with intermediate or high HBV prevalence[a] Close contacts of someone chronically infected with HBV	IVDA or hx of IVDA HIV-positive MSM Transfusion of blood products before 1986 Living in correctional facility or homeless shelter Homeless Born or brought up in country with intermediate or high HCV prevalence[a] Close contacts of someone chronically infected with HCV	IVDA or hx of IVDA Prolonged or frequent visits to areas with high incidence Residents and employees of correctional facilities, long-term care facilities, and homeless shelters Healthcare workers Medically underserved, low-income populations Alcohol abuse Foreign-born persons from areas with high incidence[b] Close contacts of someone known or suspected to have active TB

MSM men who have sex with men, *IVDA* intravenous drug abuse, *STI* sexually transmitted infection, *HBV* hepatitis B virus, *HCV* hepatitis C virus. *TB* tuberculosis

[a]Includes all countries in Africa; Asia; the Caribbean, Central, and South America; Eastern and Southern Europe; the Middle East; and the Pacific Islands

[b]Includes all countries in Africa; Asia; Eastern Europe; Latin America; and Russia

(ART). The presence of HIV does not preclude treatment with biologics. In some cases, the initiation of ART alone may allow psoriasis to regress completely [11, 13, 21–23]. In other cases, following ART initiation, psoriasis severity may become controlled to the point where treatment with a systemic agent is no longer necessary and topical therapy provides adequate disease control. For patients living with HIV who require biologic therapy to maintain control of their psoriatic disease, we recommend working closely with a HIV specialist to monitor the patient's CD4+ count and viral load.

Several guidelines including the American Academy of Dermatology (AAD)/National Psoriasis Foundation (NPF) guidelines suggest ordering HIV screening pretreatment only in select patients [1, 3]. In general, these guidelines advise utilizing clinical judgment based on a thorough patient history, clinical signs and symptoms, and/or other lab tests. Other guidelines recommend ordering baseline HIV labs in all patients prior to the initiation of biologic therapy [2, 5, 6, 8, 9]. The British Academy of Dermatology (BAD) guidelines are the most explicit regarding HIV testing [2]. They advise testing with HIV-1 and HIV-2 antibodies and HIV antigen prior to initiating biologic therapy for all patients. If testing is performed, the Centers for Disease Control and Prevention (CDC) recommends the fourth-generation combination antigen and antibody test for HIV-1 and HIV-2 as initial screening for HIV [24]. This test is ordered as a single test, commonly listed as HIV 1/2 Ag/Ab test. A positive screen is then followed by a confirmatory antibody immunodifferentiation test. If the confirmatory test is negative, then a nucleic acid test is performed to identify the presence of the p24 antigen as final confirmation. These additional steps are often performed automatically by the laboratory and then reported to the ordering provider as simply reactive or nonreactive. The penultimate confirmatory test is a quantitative polymerase chain reaction of HIV viral RNA.

BAD guidelines also advise retesting for HIV infection in any person who has symptoms or other conditions that might represent HIV infection. Additionally, they provide a weak recommendation to consider ongoing screening (annually) for HIV in those who are at increased risk. The United States Preventive Services Task Force recommends all adults ages 15–65 should be screened at least once in their lifetime. Additionally, anyone at high risk for HIV, including individuals younger than 15 and older than 65, should be screened annually independent of their psoriasis status [25]. Understanding the risk level of a given patient as well as their prior screening results is critical to allowing for a thorough assessment of a given patient prior to initiating biologic treatment. All patients with a new positive screen for HIV should immediately be referred to an HIV specialist for consideration of prompt initiation of ART as guidelines now support rapid starting of ART which has been shown to expedite the time to achieving an undetectable HIV viral load, as well as curb epidemiologic spread of HIV [26].

For patients with HIV risk factors, a thorough review of systems is prudent during routine follow-up while on biologic therapy. One should maintain a low threshold to recheck HIV serology and refer to infectious diseases if a patient develops HIV symptoms. Persons living with HIV may still be treated with biologics. Although there is limited data, a number of these patients have been successfully treated with etanercept, adalimumab, infliximab, and ustekinumab while concurrently receiving ART [27]. Several patients have also had success with secukinumab, ixekizumab, and guselkumab [28–30]. Future research is needed in this space to enhance our understanding of the risk of biologic therapies in the setting of concurrent HIV disease.

Mycobacterium Tuberculosis

TB is present worldwide. Although eight countries account for two-thirds of incident *Mycobacterium tuberculosis* (TB) cases, including India, Indonesia, China, the Philippines, Pakistan, Nigeria, Bangladesh, and South Africa, 5% of all Americans currently have latent tuberculosis infection (LTBI) [20]. Providers in the United States therefore must be aware of the risk of progression from LTBI to active tuberculosis in psoriatic patients treated with biologic and other immunosuppressive therapies. This is especially critical given the rise of drug-resistant TB and the known risk of death associated with active TB [31]. The introduction of Tumor Necrosis Factor (TNF) inhibitor therapy led to a surge in the reactivation of LTBI which highlighted this risk for dermatologists [32]. Consequently, guidelines for tuberculosis screening and monitoring were implemented by the Food and Drug Administration and specialty organizations [1, 3, 5, 6, 8–10].

Screening for LTBI prior to the initiation of a biologic agent is the most effective strategy in the prevention of progression of latent TB to active TB. Screening for all patients should include a thorough medical history, physical examination, and laboratory studies (Fig. 2.1). A thorough medical history (Table 2.2) should be performed prior to starting treatment and repeated annually to allow for an appropriate risk assessment, as patient exposure may change over time, particularly with travel. Travel to Southeast Asia, Africa, or the Western Pacific should be documented. Baseline physical examination of the left upper arm for a scar (possible prior history of a BCG vaccine) and lymph node examination are prudent in all patients prior to starting a biologic agent [33].

Risk factors for acquiring TB (Table 2.1) are distinct from risk factors for progression of LTBI to active TB while on biologic therapy (Table 2.3); this distinction is especially important in persons living with HIV or who have a history of a prior solid organ transplant given their increased risk for a poor outcome (meningitis, disseminated disease, or death) if they do develop active tuberculosis [34].

Baseline Tuberculosis Testing

Three screening tests are available for tuberculosis: the tuberculin skin test (TST) also known as purified protein derivative (PPD) and two interferon-gamma release assays (IGRAs) – QuantiFERON-TB Gold In-Tube (QFT-GIT) and T-SPOT.TB (Fig. 2.1). The TST test is read based on a classification system according to the size of the induration and the person's risk of TB infection or risk of progression to TB if infected [35]. The TST has fallen out of favor due to the require-

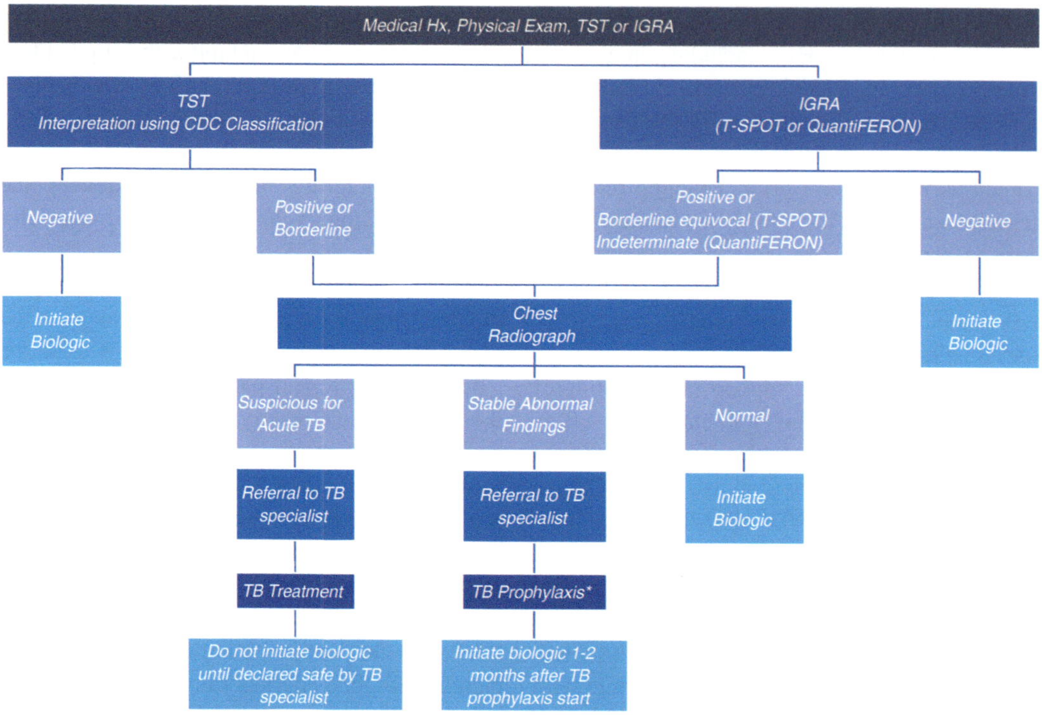

Fig. 2.1 Algorithm for diagnosis and management of tuberculosis during biologic therapy
Hx history, TST tuberculin skin test, IGRA interferon gamma release assay, CDC Centers for Disease Control and Prevention, TB tuberculosis
*Prophylaxis administration at discretion of specialist

Table 2.2 Medical history screening for tuberculosis [33]

Symptoms including ongoing cough, hemoptysis, fever, night sweats, weight loss, fatigue
History of TB, including treatment regimen and compliance with treatment
History of tuberculin skin test previously administered and associated results
History of known TB exposure
Prolonged visit to an endemic country (>3 months)
Country of origin with endemic TB status
History of BCG vaccination
Risk factors: HIV positive, IVDA, correctional facility, homeless

TB tuberculosis, *HIV* human immunodeficiency virus, *IVDA* intravenous drug abuse

ment of two visits, lesser sensitivity in comparison with IGRA, and cross-reactivity with the BCG vaccination [36]. When possible, serum studies are preferred; however, IGRAs also have limitations [37]. T-SPOT.TB appears to have a greater sensitivity when compared with QFT-GIT, but their specificities are similar [38, 39].

Notably, despite a patient having a negative TB screening test at baseline, there is still a risk of underlying TB. The false-negative rate of both TST and IGRA tests is estimated to be anywhere from 10% to 30% [38]. Snast et al. conducted a systematic review of patients with psoriasis receiving biologic therapy who developed active tuberculosis. A significant proportion (63%) had negative pretreatment screening tests. They also evaluated the type of screening test used: 56% were screened with TST, 79% IGRA, and 67% received both tests. Further, 67% of patients had no risk factors for development of primary tuberculosis. Of the 23 patients who did have a positive screening test, 78% received LTBI pro-

Table 2.3 Risk factors for progression of LTBI to active TB [34]

Diabetes mellitus
Chronic renal failure
HIV positive
Leukemia or lymphoma
Cancer of the head, neck, or lung
Cigarette smoker
Alcohol use disorder
Person who abuses drugs
Persons receiving immunosuppressive therapy
Persons infected with Mycobacterium *tuberculosis* within the past 2 years
Persons with history of untreated or inadequately treated active TB, including persons with fibrotic changes on chest radiograph consistent with prior active TB
Silicosis
History of gastrectomy or jejunoileal bypass
Weight < 90% of ideal body weight
Populations defined locally as having an increased incidence of active TB, possibly including medically underserved or low-income populations

LTBI latent tuberculosis infection, *TB* tuberculosis, *HIV* human immunodeficiency virus

phylaxis but still progressed to active TB [38]. In conclusion, providers must stay vigilant for development of active TB and educate patients to alert a healthcare professional should they develop cough, night sweats, weight loss, fever, or hemoptysis.

To date, guidelines recommend screening for TB at baseline and treating LTBI if identified [1, 3, 5, 6, 8–10]. The AAD-NPF guidelines recommend pretreatment testing with either a PPD, T-SPOT.TB, or QFT-GIT. A chest radiograph is only recommended in those with a positive TB screening test [3]. Most other worldwide guidelines recommend a chest radiograph in addition to a TB screening test at baseline, likely a response to a higher baseline incidence of TB in their respective populations [2, 3, 5, 6, 8–10].

Risk of Tuberculosis Reactivation

T helper 1 (Th1) cells have been demonstrated to play a significant role in control of *M. tuberculosis* due to their ability to increase interferon gamma [32]. Further, TNF-α is associated with the maintenance of granuloma integrity. Thus, both IL-12 and TNF-α are key players in maintaining the latent TB state.

TNF-α Inhibitors

Most data published on the risk of LTBI reactivation with biologics involves therapies in the TNF class. TB is an established risk with all TNF inhibitors, due to the integral role of TNF-α in the control of infection [2, 39]. Meta-analyses have estimated a fourfold increase of TB in those treated with TNF-α inhibitors compared to those not exposed to these drugs [39]. The risk, however, is highly dependent on the regional prevalence of TB. The monoclonal antibodies adalimumab, infliximab, and likely certolizumab carry a higher risk of reactivation than etanercept, but all TNF-α inhibitors carry significant risk [39, 40]. Those on TNFi plus methotrexate combination therapy have an even greater risk for reactivation than those on TNFi therapy alone [1, 41]. Active TB in patients on biologic therapies usually presents within the first few months of treatment. Snast et al. noted that 33% of those with active TB presented within the first 3 months of biologic therapy and 51% presented within the first 6 months. The median time to onset of active TB was shorter for the monoclonal antibodies infliximab and adalimumab, than with etanercept (3–6 months vs. >1 year) [39]. Approximately two-thirds of patients developed extrapulmonary TB reactivation and one-third disseminated disease [39]. The fatality rate ranged from 12% to 18% [39].

IL-12/23 Inhibitor

The extent of the risk of progression of latent TB to active TB in those on ustekinumab is not fully understood. Ustekinumab binds to the p40 subunit of both IL-12 and IL-23. Among 167 patients with confirmed LTBI participating in phase 3 trials, 1 patient who did not receive isoniazid prophylaxis experienced TB reactivation [42].

Another study of a national database in South Korea identified 2803 patients treated with ustekinumab. Three patients were considered to have active TB related to treatment, and none had a history of treatment of active or latent TB within 3 years prior to ustekinumab administration. The authors concluded ustekinumab did not increase the risk of TB compared with that among the general population [43]. In contrast, in the review by Snast et al. of patients with active TB treated with biologic therapy, the authors identified three cases of active TB in patients treated with ustekinumab [38]. They concluded that ustekinumab, like the TNF inhibitors, can increase the risk of progression of latent TB to active TB.

IL-23 Inhibitors

The relationship between IL-23 (a cytokine within the IL-12 family) and defense against mycobacterial infections is unclear. Data from preclinical studies suggest that the function of IL-23 in the response to TB is less important than that of other Th1-related cytokines. Analysis of pooled trial and real-world data of the three selective IL-23 inhibitors identified one case of osseous TB developing after a negative TST at screening. The patient was receiving tildrakizumab and had traveled to Asia [32]. Patients with LTBI were included in clinical trials for guselkumab and risankizumab following TB prophylaxis [32]. In one trial of risankizumab, 31 patients testing positive for LTBI were left untreated, and no cases of active TB developed [44].

IL-17 Inhibitors

T helper 17 cells are induced by IL-23. Similar to IL-23, the importance of the interleukin-17 cytokines in the defense against *Mycobacterium tuberculosis* is incompletely understood. A study using a human in vitro microgranuloma model found that the inhibition of IL-17A had little effect on TB reactivation [32]. Analysis of pooled trial and real-world data of the three available IL-17 inhibitors identified five cases of de novo active TB in patients treated with secukinumab in post-marketing surveillance and one case with ixekizumab in a country with a high TB burden. None of these cases were reported to be a reactivation. Patients with treated LTBI were not excluded from a number of phase 2, 3, and 4 secukinumab clinical trials [45]. Trials with ixekizumab also included patients with LTBI [46].

A cohort study in China of 20 patients with confirmed LTBI reported that 3 patients received prophylaxis prior to initiation of secukinumab and 17 did not. The latter were monitored with a symptom questionnaire, chest radiograph or chest computed tomography (CT), erythrocyte sedimentation rate, high-sensitivity C-reactive protein, and blood counts every 12–20 weeks. No patients developed signs of reactivation. Also of note, only one patient completed the full prophylaxis course. One participant discontinued due to anaphylaxis, and another withdrew after a persistently elevated liver transaminase level. The authors suggested that instead of mandatory chemoprophylaxis for all patients with LTBI initiated on IL-17 inhibitors, close monitoring might be a better alternative. They emphasized the importance of interdisciplinary collaboration to monitor patients, including pulmonologists and infectious (ID) disease specialists. They concluded by recommending first-line use of non-TNF-targeted biologics for patients with LTBI [47].

Gaps in knowledge still exist. These gaps will remain because the majority of randomized controlled trials are performed in the United States and western European countries where the TB prevalence is lower than in other parts of the world [39]. More studies are needed to determine the risk of LTBI reactivation. Providers should continue to screen for TB prior to initiating a biologic agent [39].

Surveillance Testing for LTBI

There is considerable debate over the utility and importance of annual testing/rescreening for LTBI in patients receiving biologic therapy [48–51].

The AAD-NPF guidelines advise yearly testing in patients at high risk. For those not at high risk, they advise screening at the discretion of the prescribing dermatologist [1]. The guidelines also emphasize the importance of screening for those on TNF-α inhibitors [1]. The Centers for Disease Control and Prevention (CDC) does not recommend rescreening of individuals during biologic therapy unless they have had a possible new exposure or have ongoing risk factors [34, 39]. The 2015 American College of Rheumatology guidelines for the treatment of rheumatoid arthritis advise rescreening only if TB risk factors are present [52]. Others feel annual TST or IGRA testing is warranted while on TNF-α inhibitor therapy [39].

Those who recommend against annual screening do so for various reasons. One study found treatment with TNF-α inhibitors decreased the sensitivity of IGRA; however IGRA still outperformed TST [39]. Another study reported annual rescreening with TST or QFT-GIT may identify 12.5% of baseline negative TNF-α patients who falsely convert at least one test. The significance of test conversion is unclear. A cohort study rescreened patients with TST, QFT-GIT, and T-SPOT.TB and found 60% converted at least one test. None of these patients were given prophylaxis and none developed active TB [53].

Given the confusion about the true risk of TB progression and the risk of false-negative testing, for IL-17 and selective IL-23 inhibitors, we recommend baseline testing, but that routine annual screening not be performed. For individuals receiving TNF-α inhibitors and ustekinumab, we concur with the AAD-NPF recommendations; baseline screening should be performed, while annual testing is recommended for those at high risk of acquiring TB or progressing from LTBI to active TB; however for individuals not at high risk, testing remains at the discretion of the provider.

Treatment of Latent Tuberculosis

Despite the well-known role of isoniazid in the treatment of latent TB, due to the extensive side effect profile, current guidelines issued by the CDC and National Tuberculosis Controllers Association favor rifamycin-based regimens over isoniazid monotherapy [54]. These regimens are shorter and have similar efficacy, favorable tolerability, and higher treatment completion rates [54]. Treatment of LTBI is usually provided in consultation with a specialist in infectious diseases. Treatment for 1–2 months is recommended prior to initiating a biologic [1]. Biologic therapy should not be initiated for those with active TB until deemed adequately treated by a specialist in TB.

Conclusion

Prior to treatment with a TNF inhibitor or ustekinumab, baseline testing for TB should be performed using an IGRA or TST. An annual risk assessment should be performed for all patients on TNF inhibitors or ustekinumab. Yearly screening with IGRA or TST should be performed for all high-risk patients (Table 2.1). For patients not at high risk, yearly testing may be considered at the prescribing clinician's discretion.

For those being treated with either the selective IL-23 inhibitors or the IL-17 inhibitors, baseline testing for TB should be performed with IGRA or TST. An annual risk assessment is also advised; however annual screening is not required.

If LTBI is identified, dermatologists should refer patients to a TB specialist, such as an infectious disease specialist or pulmonologist, for consideration of appropriate therapy. For patients with LTBI, treatment with either an IL-17 or selective IL-23 inhibitor is preferred compared with a TNF inhibitor or ustekinumab. Treatment of LTBI for 1–2 months is advised prior to biologic initiation. If active TB is identified, prompt referral to a specialist is necessary, and biologic therapy should not be initiated until deemed safe by a specialist in TB.

Hepatitis B

Hepatitis B is a vaccine-preventable viral liver infection which can cause both acute and chronic disease. The estimated prevalence of chronic hepatitis B virus (HBV) in the United States is 1.6 million persons, or roughly 0.5% of the population [55]. HBV is contracted via exposure to blood, semen, or saliva from infected persons, and those at highest risk for infection are listed in Table 2.1. Exposures in developed countries are most often a result of a sexual encounter with an infected partner, birth to an infected mother, or sharing of needles, razors, and/or toothbrushes [56].

Similar to the case of tuberculosis, although not to the same degree, the introduction of TNF-α inhibitor therapy was followed by reports of hepatitis B reactivation [57]. TNF-α plays a role in the clearance of viruses from infected hepatic cells; specifically it activates a host antiviral pathway resulting in degradation of DNA in HBV-infected cells [1, 58–60]. Additionally, while biologic therapies are not directly hepatotoxic, TNF-α inhibitors have been associated with drug-induced liver injury independent of viral hepatitis [57, 61]. Therefore, providers must be aware of the HBV status of their patients. Reactivation of latent HBV in psoriasis patients may result in cirrhosis, hepatic failure, fulminant hepatitis, and/or death [56].

Once infected with HBV, a wide range of clinical outcomes may occur. Hepatitis B serology is used to identify different phases of HBV infection including active infection, resolved infection, and immunity following vaccination as outlined in Table 2.4. In immunocompetent adults, >95% of those with symptomatic acute hepatitis B recover spontaneously [62]. Many of these patients will have a serologic pattern showing resolved HBV (Table 2.4). Other patients may become occult carriers, defined as the presence of HBV DNA in the blood of those who test negative for HBsAg (+/− anti-HBc) [63]. Occult infections are more commonly observed in pregnant women, IV drug users, and patients with concurrent hepatitis C or HIV [56]. Finally, patients with chronic HBV may have active or inactive infection, determined by HBV DNA levels, serum markers, and liver function tests.

Role of Testing

Hepatitis B screening is recommended for all patients prior to starting biologic therapy [1–3, 5, 6, 8, 10] (Fig. 2.2). Screening may uncover individuals with undiagnosed or unrecognized chronic HBV infection. Recommended screening involves a triple test for HBsAg, anti-HBs, and anti-HBc. If HBsAg returns positive, consultation with a viral hepatitis specialist such as an infectious disease specialist, gastroenterology specialist, or hepatologist is necessary prior to moving forward with biologic initiation. These patients must receive interdisciplinary management to properly assess their disease status and liver function.

Table 2.4 Interpretation of hepatitis B serologic test results [64]

Interpretation	Hepatitis B surface antigen (HBsAg)	Hepatitis B surface antibody (HBsAb, anti-HBs)	Hepatitis B core antibody (HBcAb, anti-HBc)	Hepatitis B envelope antigen (HBeAg)	Hepatitis B envelope antibody (anti-HBe)
Not immune	—	—	—	—	—
Immune due to vaccination	—	+	—	—	—
Immune due to natural infection	—	+	+	—	+ or −
Acutely infected	+	—	+	+	—
Chronically infected	+	—	+	+ or −	+ or −
Interpretation unclear[a]	—	—	+	—	+ or −

[a]Interpretation unclear, four possibilities: (1) resolved infection (most common), (2) false-positive anti-HBc (susceptible), (3) "low-level" chronic infection (occult carrier), (4) resolving acute infection

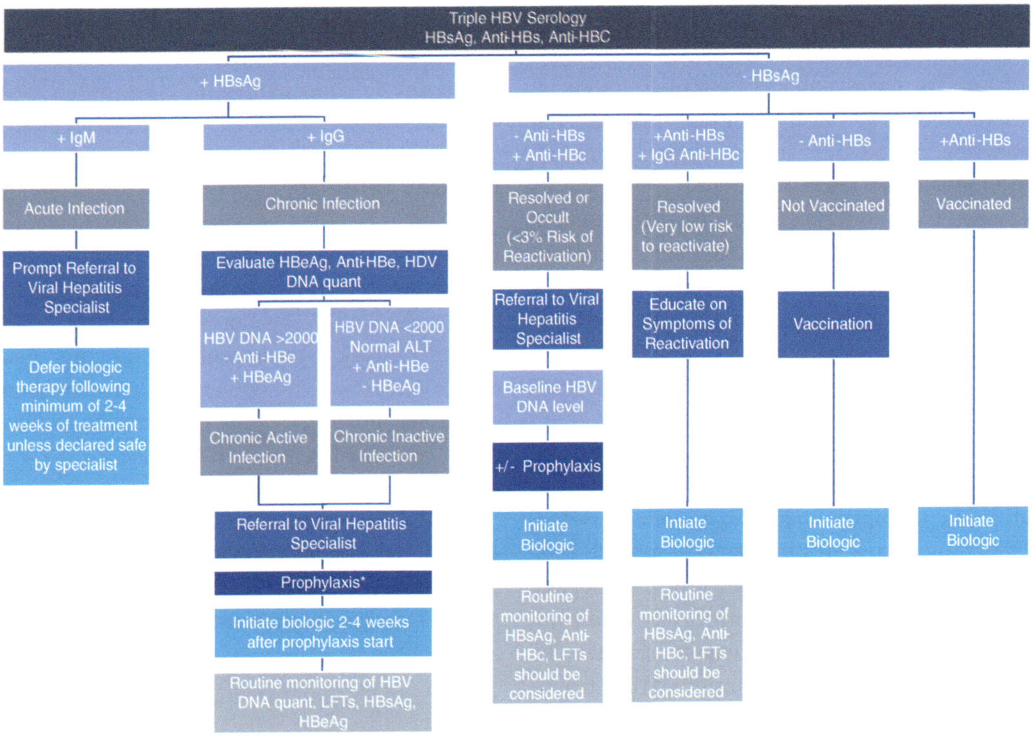

Fig. 2.2 Algorithm for diagnosis and management of hepatitis B virus during biologic therapy
HBV hepatitis B virus, LFTs liver function tests
*Prophylaxis administration for chronic inactive infection at discretion of specialist

In patients with a known history of resolved HBV or occult HBV infection (+/– anti-HBc), it is suggested to conduct pretreatment testing with HBV DNA quantification to establish a baseline [65]. For these patients, referral to ID or hepatology for evaluation prior to treatment initiation and long-term management is also advised [1]. Ongoing monitoring with HBsAg, anti-HBc, and liver function tests should be considered in patients with resolved or occult HBV [1].

If a patient is pan-negative for HBV serology, meaning they have never been vaccinated or exposed, the dermatologist should recommend vaccination and refer the patient to their primary care provider to receive the three-dose series [65]. In some cases, the vaccine may also be available at a local pharmacy or health department.

Ongoing monitoring for HBV is not required [1], but any patient who develops unexplained transaminitis during treatment with a biologic should be retested for HBV [2]. Finally, for those on biologic therapy who are unvaccinated and in a high-risk group for acquiring infection (Table 2.1), one should maintain a low threshold to recheck HBV serology.

Risk of Reactivation

Patients with chronic HBV infection receiving any immunosuppressive agent, including biologic therapy, are at risk for reactivation of HBV infection; however, this risk is not uniform. In general, criteria include a rise in HBV DNA compared to baseline and a reverse in seroconversion from HBsAg negative to HBsAg positive, if the patient was previously HBsAg negative and anti-HBc positive [62].

The risk of reactivation of HBV is minimal for patients with seropositivity for HBV core antibody receiving a biologic (1–3%) [57, 66]. Patients with chronic inactive disease are at highest risk for reactivation (14–34%) followed by occult carriers and lastly by those with resolved infection [59, 66, 67]. Those at high risk of reactivation should receive antiviral [56] medication and be carefully evaluated prior to initiating biologic therapy [59, 67]. Predictors of reactivation include HBsAg positivity, lack of prophylaxis, and young patients with a positive hepatitis B envelope antigen [66]. Baseline serum HBV DNA has not been found to be predictive of reactivation [66].

Patients should be educated regarding the risk of reactivation and advised to seek medical attention promptly should symptoms develop. Symptoms of reactivation include appetite loss, fatigue, nausea, widespread pruritus, hepatic tenderness, jaundice, dark urine, and pale stool [65]. However, HBV reactivation can also be asymptomatic [1, 67]. Thankfully, HBV reactivation is highly preventable as a result of screening and administration of prophylactic antiviral therapy [6].

TNF-α Inhibitors

A study of patients with positive HBsAg or anti-HBc receiving TNF-α inhibitors highlighted the significantly different risk for HBV reactivation among these cohorts. While 39% of positive HBsAg patients developed reactivation, only 5% of those with a positive core antibody reactivated [68]. Reactivation was more frequent in those who did not receive prophylaxis (62% vs. 23%, $P = 0.003$) [68]. Other studies have found even lower rates of reactivation following prophylaxis in positive HBsAg patients on TNF inhibitors (1–10%) [61]. In general, most cases of HBV reactivation following TNF-α inhibitors occur in nondermatological diseases [69]. Patients treated with TNF-α inhibitors have been found to have a greater risk of HBV reactivation compared to those receiving IL-17 therapy [66]. Finally, there is some evidence to suggest that etanercept may be the safest option, among the class [61].

IL-12/23 Inhibitor

Research has revealed IL-12 plays a substantial role in the body's ability to respond to hepatotropic viruses [61]. Despite this, ustekinumab has not been shown to have a substantially high risk of HBV reactivation, with rates of reactivation similar to those of TNF-α inhibitors [61]. One study identified a reactivation rate of 17.4% among patients who did not receive prophylaxis compared to 0% in those who did [70]. Other studies have concluded that ustekinumab is safe to use with positive HBV serologies, granted the patient receives prophylaxis and is comanaged by a specialist [71, 72].

IL-23 Inhibitors

Few reports of treatment with selective IL-23 inhibitors in patients with positive HBV serology exist in the literature [61, 73]. No studies or cases involving patients with positive HBV serology treated with tildrakizumab or risankizumab are available [73]. Two cases regarding guselkumab have been reported: one had a positive anti-HBc and the other positive HBsAg, anti-HBc, and hepatitis envelope antibodies. Both patients were successfully treated without reactivation [74, 75]. In a guselkumab phase 3 randomized controlled trial ($n = 739$), one case of HBV was reported [76].

IL-17 Inhibitors

In individuals with chronic liver diseases, including those resulting from viral infection, IL-17 has been found to play a role in the development of fibrosis. Thus, it is possible that inhibition of

IL-17 may confer a protective benefit from progression to cirrhosis [61]. A secukinumab study noted reactivation of HBV in 7/46 (15.2%) patients who did not receive antiviral prophylaxis [77]. Consistent with the above, patients with a positive HBsAg had significantly increased risk compared to those with a negative HBsAg and positive anti-HBc (24.0% vs. 4.17%, $P = 0.047$) [77]. Two cases involving ixekizumab and positive hepatitis B serology have been reported. The first patient was positive for HBsAg with HBV DNA (2.8 LogIU/mL), and the second was positive for anti-HBc, HBsAb, and hepatitis C virus (HCV) antibody and negative for HBsAg [78, 79]. Both patients cleared without evidence of reactivation [78, 79]. No cases or studies with brodalumab and HBV positivity have been reported, and a recent pharmacovigilance with >800 patients did not identify any cases [73].

Wu et al. recommend IL-17 inhibitors as first-line therapy followed by selective IL-23 inhibitors and then ustekinumab or a TNF-α inhibitor for patients with comorbid HBV [73]. Given the paucity of data, the effect of many of the newer biologics on hepatitis reactivation is not completely known [45], but this paradigm is reasonable until future studies clarify this further.

Treatment Regimen

Prior or current infection with HBV does not preclude someone from treatment with biologic therapy. However, close monitoring should occur in association with an infectious disease, gastroenterology, or hepatology specialist [1]. Patients may be monitored with serologies, and concurrent antiviral medication may also be prescribed.

For patients with a positive HBsAg, it is recommended to begin antiviral therapy 2–4 weeks prior to initiating a biologic, regardless of class [6]. Studies have shown that treatment with oral anti-HBV medication is effective in reducing acute exacerbations and preventing fatal complications [57].

Management of Positive Hepatitis B Core Antibody

A 2017 systematic review by Snast et al. found that 2/175 (1.1%) patients with a positive anti-HBc had viral reactivation [57]. This reflects a yearly rate of 0.32%. If a patient's serology returns positive for anti-HBc, the patient either has a resolved past infection, seropositive occult hepatitis B infection, a false-negative result, or a replicative HBsAg-negative infection (Table 2.4) [57]. Positive serology for anti-HBc does not preclude treatment with biologic therapy; however initial consultation with infectious diseases or hepatology is prudent.

Hepatitis C

In the United States, roughly 1% of the population is living with HCV [80]. Those at highest risk for infection are listed in Table 2.1. Approximately 25% of HCV infections spontaneously resolve [81]. In those who do not spontaneously clear their infection, direct acting antivirals (DAA) are available as the standard of care for those infected. DAA therapy can effectively cure >90% of individuals infected with HCV following 8–12 weeks of oral therapy [82].

Interestingly, an increased prevalence of HCV infection, but not HBV infection, has been noted in patients with psoriasis [83]. Another study found that key mediators in the pathogenesis of psoriasis are elevated in the skin of patients with HCV [84]. A series of patients with HCV and concomitant psoriasis on DAA reported that 31/37 had dramatic improvement of their psoriatic disease during DAA therapy; however 24/31 worsened after stopping therapy [85].

Role of Testing

Pretreatment screening with hepatitis C antibody tests should be completed for all patients prior to initiating a biologic [1]. Patients with a positive antibody test should be referred to their primary care provider or appropriate specialist for further work-up to assess for active infection with an HCV RNA viral load.

For those who have been treated and cured of HCV, there is no contraindication to biologic therapy, and patients can be started on treatment immediately. Of note, treated patients will have a positive antibody test for life. If a patient has a history of treated HCV, a viral load is appropriate screening to assess for a new infection, rather than a hepatitis C antibody. No routine ongoing screening for hepatitis C is recommended while on biologic therapy. Retesting with a viral load is warranted should a patient develop unexplained transaminitis while receiving biologic therapy or have a new risk of reinfection [2].

Risk of Reactivation and Treatment Regimen

Hepatitis C reactivation is extremely rare [59]. If it does occur, morbidity and mortality rates are similar to hepatitis B reactivation [59]. Studies have shown that chronic hepatitis C infection may be promoted by the upregulation of cytokines such as TNF-α [57]. Thus, it has been suggested that treatment with TNF-α inhibitors may be beneficial for patients with HCV [61, 65]. Studies of HCV-infected patients treated with TNF-α inhibitors have found viral reactivation rates of approximately 3%, which is similar to the rate of fluctuation in viral load among HCV patients [57]. Among the TNF class, etanercept is the best option considering its prior use as an adjunctive treatment in patients with HCV [61, 86, 87]. In general, most studies conclude TNF-α inhibition poses no or minimal risk for HCV reactivation [61]. In patients with HCV infection treated with ustekinumab, one of nine patients developed HCV reactivation [61, 69, 71]. No data are available on the use of selective IL-23 drugs in HCV-positive patients. In a prospective, multicenter study of patients with HCV infection treated with secukinumab, reactivation occurred in 1/14 patients who did not receive antiviral prophylaxis [4].

Patients with a history of or currently active hepatitis C may still be treated with biologic therapies; however comanagement with a viral hepatitis specialist is warranted. The goal for treatment of hepatitis C is sustained virological response, defined as the absence of detectable HCV RNA three months after completion of HCV therapy. If, however, they are not a candidate for DAA, they should be monitored with regular liver function tests (alanine aminotransaminase, aspartate aminotransferase, alkaline phosphatase, bilirubin, albumin, and platelets) in addition to HCV-RNA viral loads. Few studies are available on concurrent treatment with DAA and biologic therapies. Of the biologics utilized for psoriasis, only etanercept is mentioned in the European Association for the Study of the Liver guidelines, stating no clinically significant interaction is expected [61, 88].

Conclusion

A triple test for HBV and an HCV antibody test is recommended for all patients prior to beginning biologic therapy. For patients with seropositivity for HBV, IL-17 inhibitors may be preferred followed by selective IL-23, then IL-12/23, or a TNF inhibitor. For patients with active HCV, treatment with a DAA is recommended. Biologics can be administered concurrently provided there is multidisciplinary management with a specialist. For HCV patients, TNF inhibitors, namely, etanercept, may be considered first-line, and limited reports of patients receiving ustekinumab and secukinumab are available. All patients with HBV or HCV reactivation receiving biologic therapy should be reported via drug registries [3]. Patients should promptly seek medical attention if symptoms of reactivation develop. Multidisciplinary management is essential in this population.

Conclusion

The explosion of biologic therapy options for patients living with psoriatic disease provides us the opportunity to effectively manage patients with moderate-to-severe disease who may not have previously achieved clearance with disease-modifying antirheumatic drugs. Unfortunately, many of these drugs have not been thoroughly studied for patients with chronic infections. Thus, prescreening for TB, HBV, and HCV is necessary prior to treatment with a biologic agent. Prescreening for HIV is advised in patients with risk factors (Table 2.1). The presence of chronic infection does not preclude treatment with a biologic therapy; however, these patients must be followed closely by an interdisciplinary team to ensure the best possible outcomes.

References

1. Menter A, Strober BE, Kaplan DH, Kivelevitch D, Prater EF, Stoff B, et al. Joint AAD-NPF guidelines of care for the management and treatment of psoriasis with biologics. J Am Acad Dermatol. 2019;80(4):1029–72.
2. Smith CH, Yiu ZZN, Bale T, Burden AD, Coates LC, Edwards W, et al. British Association of Dermatologists guidelines for biologic therapy for psoriasis 2020: a rapid update. Br J Dermatol. 2020;183(4):628–37.
3. Nast A, Smith C, Spuls PI, Avila Valle G, Bata-Csörgö Z, Boonen H, et al. EuroGuiDerm guideline on the systemic treatment of Psoriasis vulgaris - Part 1: treatment and monitoring recommendations. J Eur Acad Dermatol Venereol. 2020;34(11):2461–98.
4. 2016 Addendum to the Canadian guidelines for the management of Plaque Psoriasis 2009. J Cutan Med Surg. 2016;20(5):375–431.
5. Amatore F, Villani AP, Tauber M, Viguier M, Guillot B. French guidelines on the use of systemic treatments for moderate-to-severe psoriasis in adults. J Eur Acad Dermatol Venereol. 2019;33(3):464–83.
6. Gisondi P, Altomare G, Ayala F, Bardazzi F, Bianchi L, Chiricozzi A, et al. Italian guidelines on the systemic treatments of moderate-to-severe plaque psoriasis. J Eur Acad Dermatol Venereol. 2017;31(5):774–90.
7. Kogan N, Raimondo N, Gusis SE, Izcovich A, Abarca Duran JA, Barahona-Torres L, et al. Latin American clinical practice guidelines on the systemic treatment of psoriasis SOLAPSO - Sociedad Latinoamericana de psoriasis (Latin American Psoriasis Society). Int J Dermatol. 2019;58(Suppl 1):4–28.
8. Daudén E, Puig L, Ferrándiz C, Sánchez-Carazo JL, Hernanz-Hermosa JM. Consensus document on the evaluation and treatment of moderate-to-severe psoriasis: Psoriasis Group of the Spanish Academy of Dermatology and Venereology. J Eur Acad Dermatol Venereol. 2016;30(Suppl 2):1–18.
9. Kolios AG, Yawalkar N, Anliker M, Boehncke WH, Borradori L, Conrad C, et al. Swiss S1 guidelines on the systemic treatment of psoriasis vulgaris. Dermatology. 2016;232(4):385–406.
10. Saeki H, Terui T, Morita A, Sano S, Imafuku S, Asahina A, et al. Japanese guidance for use of biologics for psoriasis (the 2019 version). J Dermatol. 2020;47(3):201–22.
11. Alpalhão M, Borges-Costa J, Filipe P. Psoriasis in HIV infection: an update. Int J STD AIDS. 2019;30(6):596–604.
12. Queirós N, Torres T. HIV-associated psoriasis. Actas Dermosifiliogr. 2018;109(4):303–11.
13. Ceccarelli M, Venanzi Rullo E, Vaccaro M, Facciolà A, d'Aleo F, Paolucci IA, et al. HIV-associated psoriasis: epidemiology, pathogenesis, and management. Dermatol Ther. 2019;32(2):e12806.
14. Mallon E, Bunker CB. HIV-associated psoriasis. AIDS Patient Care STDs. 2000;14(5):239–46.
15. Montazeri A, Kanitakis J, Bazex J. Psoriasis and HIV infection. Int J Dermatol. 1996;35(7):475–9.
16. Bartlett BL, Khambaty M, Mendoza N, Tremaine AM, Gewirtzman A, Tyring SK, et al. Dermatological management of human immunodeficiency virus (HIV). Skin Therapy Lett. 2007;12(8):1–3.
17. Goh BK, Chan RK, Sen P, Theng CT, Tan HH, Wu YJ, et al. Spectrum of skin disorders in human immunodeficiency virus-infected patients in Singapore and the relationship to CD4 lymphocyte counts. Int J Dermatol. 2007;46(7):695–9.
18. High-Impact HIV prevention: centers for disease control and prevention; 2011. Available from: https://www.cdc.gov/hiv/pdf/policies_NHPC_Booklet.pdf.
19. Hepatitis C questions and answers for health professionals centers for disease control and prevention; 2020. Available from: https://www.cdc.gov/hepatitis/hcv/hcvfaq.htm#section2.
20. Global Tuberculosis Report 2020 World Health Organization. 2020. Available from: https://apps.who.int/iris/bitstream/handle/10665/336069/9789240013131-eng.pdf.
21. Menon K, Van Voorhees AS, Bebo BF Jr, Gladman DD, Hsu S, Kalb RE, et al. Psoriasis in patients with HIV infection: from the medical board of the National Psoriasis Foundation. J Am Acad Dermatol. 2010;62(2):291–9.
22. Vittorio Luigi De Socio G, Simonetti S, Stagni G. Clinical improvement of psoriasis in an AIDS patient effectively treated with combination antiretroviral therapy. Scand J Infect Dis. 2006;38(1):74–5.
23. Duvic M, Johnson TM, Rapini RP, Freese T, Brewton G, Rios A. Acquired immunodeficiency syndrome-associated psoriasis and Reiter's syndrome. Arch Dermatol. 1987;123(12):1622–32.
24. Recommended Laboratory HIV Testing Algorithm for Serum or Plasma Specimens Centers for Disease Control and Prevention. 2014. Available from: https://www.cdc.gov/hiv/pdf/guidelines_testing_recommendedlabtestingalgorithm.pdf.
25. Owens DK, Davidson KW, Krist AH, Barry MJ, Cabana M, Caughey AB, et al. Screening for HIV infection: US preventive services task force rec-

ommendation statement. JAMA. 2019;321(23):2326–36.
26. Panel on Antiretroviral Guidelines for Adults and Adolescents. Guidelines for the use of antiretroviral agents in adults and adolescents with HIV Department of Health and Human Services. 2019. Available from: https://clinicalinfo.hiv.gov/sites/default/files/guidelines/documents/AdultandAdolescentGL.pdf.
27. Nakamura M, Abrouk M, Farahnik B, Zhu TH, Bhutani T. Psoriasis treatment in HIV-positive patients: a systematic review of systemic immunosuppressive therapies. Cutis. 2018;101(1):38;42;56.
28. Pangilinan MCG, Sermswan P, Asawanonda P. Use of anti-IL-17 monoclonal antibodies in HIV patients with Erythrodermic Psoriasis. Case Rep Dermatol. 2020;12(2):132–7.
29. Di Lernia V, Casanova DM, Garlassi E. Secukinumab in an HIV-positive patient with psoriasis. J Dtsch Dermatol Ges. 2019;17(6):646–8.
30. Bartos G, Cline A, Beroukhim K, Burrall BA, Feldman SR. Current biological therapies for use in HIV-positive patients with psoriasis: case report of gesulkumab used and review. Dermatol Online J. 2018;24(11):13030.
31. Nahid P, Mase SR, Migliori GB, Sotgiu G, Bothamley GH, Brozek JL, et al. Treatment of drug-resistant tuberculosis. An official ATS/CDC/ERS/IDSA clinical practice guideline. Am J Respir Crit Care Med. 2019;200(10):e93–e142.
32. Nogueira M, Warren RB, Torres T. Risk of tuberculosis reactivation with interleukin (IL)-17 and IL-23 inhibitors in psoriasis - time for a paradigm change. J Eur Acad Dermatol Venereol. 2021;35(4):824–34.
33. Nast A, Gisondi P, Ormerod AD, Saiag P, Smith C, Spuls PI, et al. European S3-Guidelines on the systemic treatment of psoriasis vulgaris--Update 2015--Short version--EDF in cooperation with EADV and IPC. J Eur Acad Dermatol Venereol. 2015;29(12):2277–94.
34. Mazurek GH, Jereb J, Vernon A, LoBue P, Goldberg S, Castro K. Updated guidelines for using Interferon Gamma Release Assays to detect Mycobacterium tuberculosis infection - United States, 2010. MMWR Recomm Rep. 2010;59(Rr-5):1–25.
35. Tuberculin Skin Testing Centers for Disease Control and Prevention. 2020. Available from: https://www.cdc.gov/tb/publications/factsheets/testing/skintesting.htm.
36. Ai JW, Ruan QL, Liu QH, Zhang WH. Updates on the risk factors for latent tuberculosis reactivation and their managements. Emerg Microbes Infect. 2016;5(2):e10.
37. Interferon-Gamma Release Assays (IGRAs) – Blood Tests for TB Infection Centers for Disease Control and Prevention. 2016. Available from: https://www.cdc.gov/tb/publications/factsheets/testing/igra.htm.
38. Snast I, Bercovici E, Solomon-Cohen E, Avni T, Shitenberg D, Hodak E, et al. Active tuberculosis in patients with psoriasis receiving biologic therapy: a systematic review. Am J Clin Dermatol. 2019;20(4):483–91.
39. Godfrey MS, Friedman LN. Tuberculosis and biologic therapies: anti-tumor necrosis factor-α and beyond. Clin Chest Med. 2019;40(4):721–39.
40. Rutherford AI, Patarata E, Subesinghe S, Hyrich KL, Galloway JB. Opportunistic infections in rheumatoid arthritis patients exposed to biologic therapy: results from the British Society for Rheumatology biologics register for rheumatoid arthritis. Rheumatology (Oxford). 2018;57(6):997–1001.
41. Dávila-Seijo P, Dauden E, Descalzo MA, Carretero G, Carrascosa JM, Vanaclocha F, et al. Infections in moderate to severe psoriasis patients treated with biological drugs compared to classic systemic drugs: findings from the BIOBADADERM registry. J Invest Dermatol. 2017;137(2):313–21.
42. Tsai TF, Ho V, Song M, Szapary P, Kato T, Wasfi Y, et al. The safety of ustekinumab treatment in patients with moderate-to-severe psoriasis and latent tuberculosis infection. Br J Dermatol. 2012;167(5):1145–52.
43. Cho SI, Kang S, Kim YE, Lee JY, Jo SJ. Ustekinumab does not increase tuberculosis risk: results from a national database in South Korea. J Am Acad Dermatol. 2020;82(5):1243–5.
44. Huang YW, Tsai TF. A drug safety evaluation of risankizumab for psoriasis. Expert Opin Drug Saf. 2020;19(4):395–402.
45. Wu JJ, Merola JF, Feldman SR, Menter A, Lebwohl M. Treatment of psoriasis with Secukinumab in challenging patient scenarios: a review of the available evidence. Dermatol Ther (Heidelb). 2020;10(3):351–64.
46. Mrowietz U, Riedl E, Winkler S, Xu W, Patel H, Agada N, et al. No reactivation of tuberculosis in patients with latent tuberculosis infection receiving ixekizumab: a report from 16 clinical studies of patients with psoriasis or psoriatic arthritis. J Am Acad Dermatol. 2020;83(5):1436–9.
47. Shu D, Zhang Z, Zhou EY, Ma X, Zhao Y. Is chemoprophylaxis necessary for all latent tuberculosis infection patients receiving IL-17 inhibitors? A cohort study. Dermatol Ther. 2020;33(6):e14512.
48. Duncan KO. Time to update guidelines on screening for latent tuberculosis infection in dermatologic patients being treated with tumor necrosis factor-alfa inhibitors. J Am Acad Dermatol. 2015;72(4):741–3.
49. Duncan KO, Winthrop KL. Reply to: "Comment on 'Time to update guidelines on screening for latent tuberculosis infection in dermatologic patients being treated with tumor necrosis factor-alfa inhibitors'". J Am Acad Dermatol. 2015;73(3):e125–6.
50. Doherty SD, Van Voorhees AS, Lebwohl MG, Korman NJ, Hsu S. Reply to: "Time to update guidelines on screening for latent tuberculosis infection in dermatologic patients being treated with tumor necrosis factor-alfa inhibitors". J Am Acad Dermatol. 2015;72(4):744.
51. Chirch L, Dieckhaus K, Grant-Kels JM. Reply to: "Time to update guidelines on screening for latent

tuberculosis infection in dermatologic patients being treated with tumor necrosis factor-alfa inhibitors". J Am Acad Dermatol. 2015;72(4):743.
52. Singh JA, Saag KG, Bridges SL Jr, Akl EA, Bannuru RR, Sullivan MC, et al. 2015 American College of Rheumatology Guideline for the treatment of rheumatoid arthritis. Arthritis Care Res (Hoboken). 2016;68(1):1–25.
53. Hatzara C, Hadziyannis E, Kandili A, Koutsianas C, Makris A, Georgiopoulos G, et al. Frequent conversion of tuberculosis screening tests during anti-tumour necrosis factor therapy in patients with rheumatic diseases. Ann Rheum Dis. 2015;74(10):1848–53.
54. Sterling TR, Njie G, Zenner D, Cohn DL, Reves R, Ahmed A, et al. Guidelines for the treatment of latent tuberculosis infection: recommendations from the National Tuberculosis Controllers Association and CDC, 2020. MMWR Recomm Rep. 2020;69(1):1–11.
55. Lim JK, Nguyen MH, Kim WR, Gish R, Perumalswami P, Jacobson IM. Prevalence of chronic Hepatitis B virus infection in the United States. Am J Gastroenterol. 2020;115(9):1429–38.
56. Motaparthi K, Stanisic V, Van Voorhees AS, Lebwohl MG, Hsu S. From the Medical Board of the National Psoriasis Foundation: recommendations for screening for hepatitis B infection prior to initiating anti-tumor necrosis factor-alfa inhibitors or other immunosuppressive agents in patients with psoriasis. J Am Acad Dermatol. 2014;70(1):178–86.
57. Snast I, Atzmony L, Braun M, Hodak E, Pavlovsky L. Risk for hepatitis B and C virus reactivation in patients with psoriasis on biologic therapies: a retrospective cohort study and systematic review of the literature. J Am Acad Dermatol. 2017;77(1):88–97.e5.
58. Calabrese LH, Zein NN, Vassilopoulos D. Hepatitis B virus (HBV) reactivation with immunosuppressive therapy in rheumatic diseases: assessment and preventive strategies. Ann Rheum Dis. 2006;65(8):983–9.
59. Bonifati C, Lora V, Graceffa D, Nosotti L. Management of psoriasis patients with hepatitis B or hepatitis C virus infection. World J Gastroenterol. 2016;22(28):6444–55.
60. Loomba R, Liang TJ. Hepatitis B reactivation associated with immune suppressive and biological modifier therapies: current concepts, management strategies, and future directions. Gastroenterology. 2017;152(6):1297–309.
61. Piaserico S, Messina F, Russo FP. Managing psoriasis in patients with HBV or HCV infection: practical considerations. Am J Clin Dermatol. 2019;20(6):829–45.
62. Terrault NA, Lok ASF, McMahon BJ, Chang KM, Hwang JP, Jonas MM, et al. Update on prevention, diagnosis, and treatment of chronic hepatitis B: AASLD 2018 hepatitis B guidance. Hepatology. 2018;67(4):1560–99.
63. Raimondo G, Locarnini S, Pollicino T, Levrero M, Zoulim F, Lok AS. Update of the statements on biology and clinical impact of occult hepatitis B virus infection. J Hepatol. 2019;71(2):397–408.
64. Interpretation of Hepatitis B serologic test results Centers for Disease Control and Prevention, Division of Viral Hepatitis. 2020 [Available from: https://www.cdc.gov/hepatitis/hbv/pdfs/serologicchartv8.pdf.
65. Poelman SM, Keeling CP, Metelitsa AI. Practical guidelines for managing patients with psoriasis on biologics: an update. J Cutan Med Surg. 2019;23(1_suppl):3s–12s.
66. Chiu HY, Chiu YM, Chang Liao NF, Chi CC, Tsai TF, Hsieh CY, et al. Predictors of hepatitis B and C virus reactivation in patients with psoriasis treated with biologic agents: a 9-year multicenter cohort study. J Am Acad Dermatol 2019.
67. Abramson A, Menter A, Perrillo R. Psoriasis, hepatitis B, and the tumor necrosis factor-alpha inhibitory agents: a review and recommendations for management. J Am Acad Dermatol. 2012;67(6):1349–61.
68. Pérez-Alvarez R, Díaz-Lagares C, García-Hernández F, Lopez-Roses L, Brito-Zerón P, Pérez-de-Lis M, et al. Hepatitis B virus (HBV) reactivation in patients receiving tumor necrosis factor (TNF)-targeted therapy: analysis of 257 cases. Medicine. 2011;90(6):359–71.
69. Navarro R, Vilarrasa E, Herranz P, Puig L, Bordas X, Carrascosa JM, et al. Safety and effectiveness of ustekinumab and antitumour necrosis factor therapy in patients with psoriasis and chronic viral hepatitis B or C: a retrospective, multicentre study in a clinical setting. Br J Dermatol. 2013;168(3):609–16.
70. Ting SW, Chen YC, Huang YH. Risk of Hepatitis B reactivation in patients with psoriasis on Ustekinumab. Clin Drug Investig. 2018;38(9):873–80.
71. Chiu HY, Chen CH, Wu MS, Cheng YP, Tsai TF. The safety profile of ustekinumab in the treatment of patients with psoriasis and concurrent hepatitis B or C. Br J Dermatol. 2013;169(6):1295–303.
72. Siegel SAR, Winthrop KL, Ehst BD, Ortega LA. Ustekinumab use in patients with severe psoriasis co-infected with hepatitis B and/or C. Br J Dermatol. 2019;180(5):1232–3.
73. Thatiparthi A, Martin A, Liu J, Egeberg A, Wu JJ. Biologic treatment algorithms for moderate-to-severe psoriasis with comorbid conditions and special populations: a review. Am J Clin Dermatol. 2021;22(4):425–42.
74. Song EJ, Whitman P, Samsel J. The use of ustekinumab and guselkumab in a pediatric psoriasis patient with active hepatitis B infection. JAAD Case Rep. 2021;8:37–9.
75. Duncan JR, Orlowski TJ, Elewski BE. Safety of guselkumab in hepatitis B virus infection. Dermatol Online J. 2019;25(10):13030.
76. Mease PJ, Rahman P, Gottlieb AB, Kollmeier AP, Hsia EC, Xu XL, et al. Guselkumab in biologic-naive patients with active psoriatic arthritis (DISCOVER-2): a double-blind, randomised, placebo-controlled phase 3 trial. Lancet. 2020;395(10230):1126–36.
77. Chiu HY, Hui RC, Huang YH, Huang RY, Chen KL, Tsai YC, et al. Safety profile of Secukinumab in treatment of patients with psoriasis and concurrent

Hepatitis B or C: a multicentric prospective cohort study. Acta Derm Venereol. 2018;98(9):829–34.
78. Koike Y, Fujiki Y, Higuchi M, Fukuchi R, Kuwatsuka S, Murota H. An interleukin-17 inhibitor successfully treated a complicated psoriasis and psoriatic arthritis patient with hepatitis B virus infection and end-stage kidney disease on hemodialysis. JAAD Case Rep. 2019;5(2):150–2.
79. Lora V, Graceffa D, De Felice C, Morrone A, Bonifati C. Treatment of severe psoriasis with ixekizumab in a liver transplant recipient with concomitant hepatitis B virus infection. Dermatol Ther. 2019;32(3):e12909.
80. Hofmeister MG, Rosenthal EM, Barker LK, Rosenberg ES, Barranco MA, Hall EW, et al. Estimating prevalence of Hepatitis C virus infection in the United States, 2013-2016. Hepatology. 2019;69(3):1020–31.
81. Grebely J, Prins M, Hellard M, Cox AL, Osburn WO, Lauer G, et al. Hepatitis C virus clearance, reinfection, and persistence, with insights from studies of injecting drug users: towards a vaccine. Lancet Infect Dis. 2012;12(5):408–14.
82. Hepatitis C. Guidance 2018 update: AASLD-IDSA recommendations for testing, managing, and treating Hepatitis C virus infection. Clin Infect Dis. 2018;67(10):1477–92.
83. Cohen AD, Weitzman D, Birkenfeld S, Dreiher J. Psoriasis associated with hepatitis C but not with hepatitis B. Dermatology. 2010;220(3):218–22.
84. Chun K, Afshar M, Audish D, Kabigting F, Paik A, Gallo R, et al. Hepatitis C may enhance key amplifiers of psoriasis. J Eur Acad Dermatol Venereol. 2017;31(4):672–8.
85. Cacciola I, Borgia F, Filomia R, Pitrone C, Franzè MS, Alibrandi A, et al. Outcome of cutaneous psoriasis in hepatitis C virus-infected patients treated with direct-acting antiviral therapy. J Viral Hepat. 2020;27(3):333–7.
86. Zein NN. Etanercept as an adjuvant to interferon and ribavirin in treatment-naive patients with chronic hepatitis C virus infection: a phase 2 randomized, double-blind, placebo-controlled study. J Hepatol. 2005;42(3):315–22.
87. Chularojanamontri L, Nimanong S, Wongpraparut C, Silpa-Archa N, Chaiyabutr C, Charoenpipatsin N. How do we treat psoriasis patients with hepatitis C infections in real-world situations? A retrospective analysis of 34 patients. J Dermatolog Treat. 2021;32(3):321–7.
88. EASL recommendations on treatment of hepatitis C: final update of the series(☆). J Hepatol. 2020;73(5):1170–218.

TNF-Alpha Class of Biologic Agents in Psoriatic Disease

3

Mark Weingarten and Mark Lebwohl

Introduction

This chapter reviews the efficacy and safety of tumor necrosis factor-alpha (TNF-α) antagonists in the treatment of psoriasis and psoriatic arthritis. It further delineates nuances in individual medication profiles to consider in the selection of a treatment regimen.

Efficacy of TNF-α Antagonists in the Treatment of Psoriasis

Certolizumab pegol efficacy for psoriasis has been documented by the CIMPASI I, CIMPASI II, and CIMPACT phase 3 trials. Pooled analysis of 850 patients from these studies analyzed patients treated with 400 mg, 200 mg, or placebo control every 2 weeks. At 16 weeks, 80.1% of the 400 mg experimental group surpassed the PASI 75 marker (76%, 67%, 7% for 400 mg, 200 mg, and placebo in CIMPASI 1; 83%, 81%, and 12%, respectively, for CIMPASI 2) [1]. Concurrently, 63.7% of this treatment group in pooled analysis reached a physician global assessment (PGA) of 0/1, a qualitative marker of "clear" or "almost clear" involvement. Outcomes of the pooled 200 mg experimental group were robust even as they were slightly less impressive. 74.5% and 54.6% achieved PASI 75 reduction and 0/1 PGA, respectively. In contrast, only 7.5% and 2.8% of the control groups achieved similar respective outcomes. This difference in improvement applied regardless of previous exposure to biologic therapy [1, 2].

The CIMPACT trial is further notable because it included a large-scale comparison of certolizumab pegol efficacy to that of etanercept (50 mg, twice weekly) at 12 weeks. In contrast to the 66.7 and 61.3% who achieved PASI 75 among the certolizumab pegol groups (400 mg; 200 mg) at week 12, 53.3% of the etanercept group achieved PASI 75 at week 12 even as baseline disease characteristics between the groups were similar; PGA 0/1 achievement rates were statistically greater among the 400 mg certolizumab pegol group (50.3%), while non-inferior among the 200 mg certolizumab pegol group (39.8%) when compared to etanercept (39.2%). Combined, the CIMPACT trial supports increased efficacy of certolizumab pegol in comparison to etanercept [3]. Simultaneously, the degree of increased efficacy of certolizumab pegol against etanercept should be appreciated in the context of data associating etanercept with slightly fewer adverse events as discussed below [3].

M. Weingarten
Icahn School of Medicine at Mount Sinai Hospital, New York, NY, USA

M. Lebwohl (✉)
Department of Dermatology, Icahn School of Medicine at Mount Sinai Hospital, New York, NY, USA

N. Brownstone et al. (eds.), *Biologic Therapy for Psoriasis*, Updates in Clinical Dermatology,
https://doi.org/10.1007/978-3-030-92938-1_3

Etanercept's efficacy at 50 mg twice weekly was also tested in comparison to ixekizumab in the UNCOVER-2 and UNCOVER-3 phase 3 trials. At 12 weeks, etanercept patients in UNCOVER-2 and UNCOVER-3 displayed PASI 75 in 41.6% and 53.4% as well as PGA 0/1 in 36.0% and 41.6% in the two trials, respectively [4]. In a separate open-label study, PASI 75 rate at week 12 among etanercept patients following failed apremilast therapy was identical to those of the UNCOVER-2 trial at 41.6% [5]. In a similar examination of etanercept use after failing to respond to adalimumab, PASI 75 rates were 47.5% among those who had adalimumab antibodies and 50% of those who didn't. PGA 0/1 was 45% and 35% among those respective groups, a difference not found to bear statistical significance [6]. While adalimumab antibodies were not found to limit treatment efficacy in this study, its design and sample size justify further investigation of this phenomenon. In other studies, etanercept's efficacy in the presence of antibodies developed against it was found to be unique in this regard. While patients develop antibodies to etanercept as they do to adalimumab, anti-etanercept antibodies have not been found to neutralize drug efficacy [7, 8]. In contrast, anti-adalimumab antibodies were found in multiple studies to diminish drug efficacy [9–11].

While adalimumab's efficacy can be weakened by the presence of antibodies, a meta-analysis found adalimumab to be more efficacious than etanercept in achieving PASI 90 in the absence of trials that directly compare the two [12]. In the recent BESURE trials of 478 patients comparing the use of bimekizumab to adalimumab, the latter was found to exhibit a PASI 75 of 31.4% at week 4 and a PASI 90 of 47.7% and IGA 0/1 of 57.2 at week 16 [13]. A large phase 3 trial of patients in China found that 77.8% of adalimumab 40 mg Q2 weeks achieved PASI 75 at week 12 compared to 11.5% in placebo; PGA 0/1 was 80.5% in the adalimumab-treated subjects compared to 14.9% in the placebo arm [14]. In the phase 3 BELIEVE trial performed a decade earlier in which patients were given an 80 mg initial dose of adalimumab followed by 40 mg every other week, 70.9% achieved PASI 75 at week 16 on monotherapy, while 64.8% achieved that endpoint with adalimumab and topical calcipotriol or betamethasone. No statistical difference was found between the two groups [15]. Although the class TNF-α inhibitors have been associated with increased cancer risk as described below, even as the risk for adalimumab has not been clearly established [16–18], a randomized controlled trial spanning 15 European countries with withdrawal, retreatment, and long-term extension groups in children found that at week 16, 57.9% of those given 0.8 mg/kg achieved PASI 75 compared with 43.6% of those given 0.4 mg/kg and 32.4% of those given methotrexate. After a 52-week long-term extension, 86.1% of those given 0.8 mg/kg after 16 weeks methotrexate attained PASI 75, followed by 72.2% of those given 0.8 mg/kg throughout and 47.2% of those given 0.4 mg/kg followed by 0.4 or 0.8 at week 16 [19]. Long-term use of adalimumab is associated with greater efficacy, with one randomized controlled trial finding that among those who had obtained PASI 75 at 32 weeks, 28% of patients who replaced adalimumab with placebo between weeks 32 and 52 significantly lost adequate response compared to only 5% among those who continued the adalimumab for the duration of the 52 weeks [9]. Adalimumab has also been found in open-label studies to be efficacious following unsuccessful etanercept regimens just as the reverse phenomenon as described above [20–22].

Efficacy of TNF-α Antagonists in the Treatment of Psoriatic Arthritis

Certolizumab pegol efficacy for psoriatic arthritis was demonstrated in the 4-year RAPID-PSA phase 3 trial. ACR20 improvement was achieved by 58% of subjects in the certolizumab pegol 400 Q4W arm and 52% in the 200 Q2W arm in comparison to 24% of placebo-treated subjects at week 12; ACR50 was likewise achieved by 42.1% as opposed to 12.5% in the placebo arm by week 24. At 48 weeks, 78.7% of patients achieved Psoriasis Area and Severity Index (PASI) 75, 28.5% achieved Disease Activity in Psoriatic Arthritis (DAPSA) complete remission, and 37.7% achieved DAPSA low disease activity. These numbers were maintained and improved to the study's conclusion at week 216. 79.6% of patients achieved PASI 75, 44% experienced DAPSA remission by the end of the 4 years, while 32% reached DAPSA low disease state. No significant findings in the progression of joint damage were noted across the duration of treatment course. These results were relatively independent of previous TNF-α exposure [23].

Direct comparisons between adalimumab, etanercept, and infliximab (albeit excluding certolizumab pegol) found them to be relatively similar in efficacy for psoriatic arthritis. ACR20 at 12 months was 70% in adalimumab, 72% for etanercept, and 75% for infliximab. Interestingly, etanercept was particularly efficacious among patients who complained of deficits in articular function, while adalimumab was linked with greater improvements for those with skin involvement [24]. While this data may be confounded by the variability of concurrent methotrexate usage, similar results were obtained in a separate meta-analysis [25]. Independent comparisons that added golimumab further buttressed and extended the lack of novelty between medications with respect to their relation to ACR50 at 24 weeks [26].

Independent studies of both adalimumab and golimumab for psoriatic arthritis were comparable to these results at shorter intervals. In the SELECT-PsA-1 double-blind phase 3 trial involving 45 countries, 65% of the 429 patients who received adalimumab 40 mg every 2 weeks experienced ACR 20% improvement at 12 weeks compared to 36.2 weeks with placebo [27].

The GO-VIBRANT phase 3 randomized controlled trial compared golimumab given 2 mg/kg at weeks 0 and 4 and then every 8 weeks to placebo. ACR20 at 14 weeks was 75.1% for the experimental group as opposed to 21.8% achieved in the placebo control. 59.5% of the experimental group achieved PASI 75 at 14 weeks in comparison to 12.5% of the placebo control group among those who did not use methotrexate at baseline; PASI 75 among those that did were 59.5% and 14.1%, respectively. Of note, those found with antidrug antibodies lacked high titers or expressed the same robust response although this ancillary finding requires further investigation [28]. Analysis of GO-VIBRANT at 52 weeks found a consistent 76.8% of patients in the golimumab group and 77.0% in the placebo- crossover group achieved an ACR20 response, 58.1% and 53.6%, respectively, achieved an ACR50 response, and 38.6% and 33.9%, respectively, achieved an ACR70 response. PASI75 response rates were 71.9% in the golimumab group and 60.6% in the placebo- crossover group [29]. In comparing the GO VIBRANT Trial to the GO REVEAL study conducted nearly a decade prior, the latter had found that at 14 weeks ACR 20 was 51% for a 50 mg golimumab regimen, 45% for a 100 mg regimen, and 9% for placebo; PASI 75 scores were 40% in 50 mg, 58% in 100 mg, 3% in placebo [30]. Week 52 results for GO REVEAL demonstrated that efficacy was maintained and improved, with ACR20 of 66% for the 50 mg group (including those who received 100mg starting at week 16), 67% for the 100 mg group, and 71% for subjects in the placebo group who crossed over to 50 mg at week 16 or week 24. PASI 75 scores were 62.4%, 68.5%, and 48.1%, respectively [31].

Safety Profiles of TNF-α Inhibitors in the Treatment of Psoriasis and Psoriatic Arthritis

TNF-α inhibitors have been associated with an increased risk of developing infection and malignancy. Any patient with active malignancy or serious infection should not be placed on one of these drugs, and caution should be exercised before prescribing a TNF-α inhibitor in a patient with prominent history of either. TNF-α inhibitors have been shown to exacerbate demyelinating diseases and are contraindicated in patients with multiple sclerosis [32].

Safety concerns may be further stratified by timing from medication commencement, with the initial period of highest concern. They have also been investigated by patient age. A retrospective observational study found no age-related difference in efficacy or adverse events that could render the elderly (those over 65) particularly vulnerable to the TNF antibody class when compared with adult counterparts. In fact, the elderly experienced more adverse events when on systemic treatment for psoriasis (acitretin, cyclosporin, and methotrexate) in comparison to biologics (including adalimumab, certolizumab pegol, etanercept, golimumab) [33].

Patient risk of developing infection is particularly increased among those on concurrent regimens of immunosuppressants, which themselves predispose to infection. These include methotrexate and corticosteroids. Nevertheless, the ambiguity concerning the risks (and efficacies) subsequently posed by TNF-α inhibitors in these patients is largely confined to those suffering from rheumatoid arthritis who commonly are on concurrent immunosuppressive medications. Reduction of steroid therapy in such patients has been associated with a decrease in infection rates [34]. In contrast, the phase 3 studies of TNF-α inhibitors for psoriasis described here are predominantly monotherapy trials unless otherwise noted, thereby eliminating this particular concern.

Infections can present as viral, bacterial, or fungal etiology. Tuberculosis, legionella, and listeria infection have been reported. Histoplasmosis, coccidioidomycosis, candidiasis, aspergillosis, blastomycosis, and pneumocystis are the predominant fungal infections recorded and described on black box warnings for the entire TNF-α class. Despite this broad indictment, nuances exist between TNF-α inhibitors to distinguish their safety profile.

In a 2011 Cochrane review which studied the safety of TNF-α across all approved indications, certolizumab pegol was found to have a significantly higher risk of infection among the TNF-α agents studied. Certolizumab pegol was deemed significantly associated with severe adverse events requiring hospitalization (other than infection) in comparison to placebo. In comparison with the other agents, certolizumab pegol was more implicated in such events than adalimumab, which in turn had a higher association than did golimumab [35]. However, this data concerning adverse events is mitigated by subsequent sensitivity analysis adjusted for dose that found no statistical significance between them. Moreover, as noted above, the association between certolizumab pegol and infections requires qualification. In contrast to assumptions that TNF-α inhibitor side effects are independent of the disease process involved, they exhibited a greater association with noninfectious adverse events among patients with psoriasis and ankylosing spondylitis, while their association with infection was far more relevant to rheumatoid or psoriatic arthritis than to psoriasis in comparison to controls.

In more recent studies of psoriasis patients treated with certolizumab pegol, the percent who experienced infections among the placebo group was greater than those in the 200 mg group, while less than that among the 400 mg group. Serious adverse effects other than infection were similar between 400 mg experimental and placebo control, both of which were significantly greater than in the 200 mg experimental group [2]. For psoriatic arthritis patients treated with certolizumab pegol, infections remain of prominent note to the monitoring physician. While no placebo group is available for comparison, 6% of patients on certolizumab pegol for 4 years experienced a serious infection, most commonly pneumonia [23].

Certolizumab's role as the most highly associated with infection among the TNF-α inhibitors discussed has not been proven to extend to tuberculosis. In the most recent large analysis of phase 3 trials, only 1 case of tuberculosis was reported among 995 patients who received at least 1 dose of certolizumab pegol [36]. The comprehensive nature of this study and reassuring nature of its results is somewhat mitigated by the fact that the patients studied were from Europe and North America. Tuberculosis rates among patients on certolizumab pegol regimens in Asian countries where the disease is more prevalent were found to be similar to those of the general population [37]. Nevertheless, the overall concerns of TB in conjunction with TNF-α antagonists use is concerning. One pooled study found a total of 45 TB cases occurred among 7912 patients treated with

TNF-α antagonists and only 3 cases developed out of 3967 [38]. Concern for TB infection warrants continued TB testing prior to treatment onset. Patients with latent tuberculosis should be treated prior to starting TNF-α antagonist therapy.

Beyond the strong efficacy reports, certolizumab pegol is of particular interest to pregnant patients. In contrast to other anti-TNF therapies, certolizumab pegol has minimal transfer across the placenta because it lacks the IgG Fc. As a result, it is unable to bind the neonatal Fc receptor. Therefore, while TNF-α antagonists have not been proven to pose a risk to fetal or maternal health, a greater inherent risk is possible [39–41]. Certolizumab pegol remains an excellent option for pregnant as well as nursing patients with psoriasis [42].

Certolizumab pegol's risk profile is further important to the many patients suffering from both psoriasis and Crohn's disease. Certolizumab pegol and adalimumab are efficacious in the treatment of Crohn's and therefore would be preferred in such cases [43, 44]. In contrast, etanercept was independently shown to have no benefit in improving Crohn's [45].

Even as it is not used in cases of Crohn's, etanercept has a relatively low infectious risk profile as well as the lowest tuberculosis rates among the TNF blockers [46]. When compared independently to placebo in a separate integrated analysis of different studies for psoriasis alone and psoriatic arthritis, there were comparable rates of serious adverse events and infection between placebo and etanercept groups. This included both short- and long-term treatment data points regardless of differences in dose [47, 48]. Adverse events tended to decrease in prevalence over time as noted with respect to certolizumab pegol. Notable adverse event among the UNCOVER trials was grade 3 neutropenia among four patients [4]. When directly compared with certolizumab pegol in the CIMPACT trial, etanercept had slightly less total adverse events, but infection rates were relatively similar [3].

A higher rate of non-melanoma skin cancer was documented among the etanercept groups in major analyses [47, 48]. This data must be considered in the context of multiple patients with prior psoralen and ultraviolet A exposure (PUVA) [49], prior immunosuppressant use [50], and a larger overall risk in squamous cell carcinoma among psoriasis patients that defies attribution to a particular therapy [51]. Studies of other malignancy rates found no difference between etanercept and placebo, or a greater prevalence in cancers among psoriatic arthritis and psoriasis patients on etanercept in comparison to that of the general population [48]. Cancer rates in etanercept among psoriasis patients are lower than that of infliximab or adalimumab.

Similarly, adalimumab has relatively low risk regarding its rate of adverse events, infection, and malignancy among patients treated for psoriasis. In the study comparing adalimumab, etanercept, and infliximab, adalimumab had the lowest rate of adverse events (6%) compared with etanercept (17%) and with infliximab (23%). Similarly, the major studies referenced above documented no incidence of demyelinating disease or tuberculosis among adalimumab patients, with the exception of the study conducted in China where tuberculosis remains endemic [13, 14, 24]. The BE SURE trial of adalimumab found only 1 serious infection, 1 malignancy, and 5 serious adverse events among 159 patients [13]. The study conducted in China found that 3.5% of patients experienced serious adverse events, and 1.2% [4] experienced serious infection. No cancers were found in this study [14].

In review of adalimumab's safety with respect to its role in treating psoriatic arthritis, the BELIEVE phase 3 trial found one incidence of pneumonia, one staphylococcal infection, and one lymphoma among the adalimumab experimental group. The lymphoma was found 7 weeks after commencement of the treatment regimen, and an elevated lymphocyte count had been observed at initial screening. It was therefore deemed likely unrelated to the treatment course. Single cases of pneumonia, herpes zoster, squamous cell carcinoma (diagnosed at 2 weeks), and malignant melanoma (diagnosed at 7 weeks) were each found among members of the experimental group that combined adalimumab with topical betamethasone/calcipotriol [15]. A case of herpes zoster was also found among the pediatric population treated with adalimumab [19]. A separate study found that both rates of adverse events (3.7%) and serious infections (0.7%) among adalimumab patients were comparable to those while on placebo regimens. Moreover, the same study found no herpes zoster or TB. While the study was notable for the degree to which adalimumab was associated with hepatic disorders (15.6%), rates of grade ALT and AST elevations among the experimental group were less than those of control [27]. 0.7% were diagnosed with cancer, and 2.3% experienced neutropenia.

Adverse effects reported in patients on golimumab regimens for psoriatic arthritis are comparable to those described for the other medications above. In the GO-VIBRANT trials, there were no findings of tuberculosis, noninfectious encephalomyelitis, or cancer in experimental group throughout the first 24 weeks. One pneumonia was reported, as were ALT elevations within 2x normal limit [28]. At 1 year, two incidents of cancer (one gastric and one colon) were reported, along with two additional cases of pneumonia and two cases of tuberculosis [29].

Conclusion

In conclusion, a vast amount of phase 3, multicenter trials of TNF-α antagonists have established their efficacy in the treatment of moderate-to-severe psoriasis and, along with golimumab, in the treatment of psoriatic arthritis. These trials found that adalimumab and certolizumab pegol have higher efficacy than etanercept in the treatment of psoriasis, a distinction that is less prominent in studies of both short- and long-term administration of these medications in cases of psoriatic arthritis. Relative decreases of etanercept efficacy in psoriasis compared to certolizumab pegol and adalimumab must be considered in the context of etanercept's better safety profile. The nuanced benefits and deficiencies presented here are important to take into consideration for high-quality patient care when using TNF-α inhibitors.

References

1. Gottlieb AB, Blauvelt A, Thaçi D, et al. Certolizumab pegol for the treatment of chronic plaque psoriasis: Results through 48 weeks from 2 phase 3, multicenter, randomized, double-blinded, placebo-controlled studies (CIMPASI-1 and CIMPASI-2). J Am Acad Dermatol. 2018;79(2):302–314.e6. https://doi.org/10.1016/j.jaad.2018.04.012.
2. Blauvelt A, Reich K, Lebwohl M, et al. Certolizumab pegol for the treatment of patients with moderate-to-severe chronic plaque psoriasis: pooled analysis of week 16 data from three randomized controlled trials. J Eur Acad Dermatol Venereol. 2019;33(3):546–52. https://doi.org/10.1111/jdv.15258.
3. Lebwohl M, Blauvelt A, Paul C, et al. Certolizumab pegol for the treatment of chronic plaque psoriasis: Results through 48 weeks of a phase 3, multicenter, randomized, double-blind, etanercept- and placebo-controlled study (CIMPACT). J Am Acad Dermatol. 2018;79(2):266–276.e5. https://doi.org/10.1016/j.jaad.2018.04.013.
4. Griffiths CE, Reich K, Lebwohl M, et al. Comparison of ixekizumab with etanercept or placebo in moderate-to-severe psoriasis (UNCOVER-2 and UNCOVER-3): results from two phase 3 randomised trials. Lancet. 2015;386(9993):541–51. https://doi.org/10.1016/S0140-6736(15)60125-8.
5. Bagel J, Samad AS, Stolshek BS, et al. Open-label study to evaluate the efficacy of Etanercept treatment in subjects with moderate to severe plaque psoriasis who have failed therapy with apremilast. J Drugs Dermatol. 2018;17(10):1078–82.
6. Bagel J, Tyring S, Rice KC, et al. Open-label study of etanercept treatment in patients with moderate-to-severe plaque psoriasis who lost a satisfactory response to adalimumab. Br J Dermatol. 2017;177(2):411–8. https://doi.org/10.1111/bjd.15381.
7. Papp KA, Tyring S, Lahfa M, et al. A global phase III randomized controlled trial of etanercept in psoriasis: safety, efficacy, and effect of dose reduction. Br J Dermatol. 2005;152(6):1304–12. https://doi.org/10.1111/j.1365-2133.2005.06688.x.
8. Leonardi C, Strober B, Gottlieb AB, et al. Long-term safety and efficacy of etanercept in patients with psoriasis: an open-label study. J Drugs Dermatol. 2010;9(8):928–37.
9. Menter A, Tyring SK, Gordon K, et al. Adalimumab therapy for moderate to severe psoriasis: a randomized, controlled phase III trial. J Am Acad Dermatol. 2008;58(1):106–15. https://doi.org/10.1016/j.jaad.2007.09.010.
10. Takahashi H, Tsuji H, Ishida-Yamamoto A, Iizuka H. Plasma trough levels of adalimumab and infliximab in terms of clinical efficacy during the treatment of psoriasis. J Dermatol. 2013;40(1):39–42. https://doi.org/10.1111/j.1346-8138.2012.01679.x.
11. Mahil SK, Arkir Z, Richards G, Lewis CM, Barker JN, Smith CH. Predicting treatment response in pso-

riasis using serum levels of adalimumab and etanercept: a single-Centre, cohort study. Br J Dermatol. 2013;169(2):306–13. https://doi.org/10.1111/bjd.12341.
12. Sbidian E, Chaimani A, Afach S, et al. Systemic pharmacological treatments for chronic plaque psoriasis: a network meta-analysis. Cochrane Database Syst Rev. 2020;1(1):CD011535. Published 2020 Jan 9. https://doi.org/10.1002/14651858.CD011535.pub3.
13. Warren RB, Blauvelt A, Bagel J, et al. Bimekizumab versus Adalimumab in Plaque Psoriasis. N Engl J Med. 2021;385(2):130–41. https://doi.org/10.1056/NEJMoa2102388.
14. Cai L, Gu J, Zheng J, et al. Efficacy and safety of adalimumab in Chinese patients with moderate-to-severe plaque psoriasis: results from a phase 3, randomized, placebo-controlled, double-blind study. J Eur Acad Dermatol Venereol. 2017;31(1):89–95. https://doi.org/10.1111/jdv.13746.
15. Thaçi D, Ortonne JP, Chimenti S, et al. A phase IIIb, multicentre, randomized, double-blind, vehicle-controlled study of the efficacy and safety of adalimumab with and without calcipotriol/betamethasone topical treatment in patients with moderate to severe psoriasis: the BELIEVE study. Br J Dermatol. 2010;163(2):402–11. https://doi.org/10.1111/j.1365-2133.2010.09791.x.
16. Humira (adalimumab) [prescribing information]. North Chicago, IL: AbbVie Inc; 2021.
17. Alvisi P, Dipasquale V, Barabino A, et al. Infections and malignancies risks related to TNF-α-blocking agents in pediatric inflammatory bowel diseases. Expert Rev Gastroenterol Hepatol. 2019;13(10):957–61. https://doi.org/10.1080/17474124.2019.1663173.
18. Dulai PS, Thompson KD, Blunt HB, Dubinsky MC, Siegel CA. Risks of serious infection or lymphoma with anti-tumor necrosis factor therapy for pediatric inflammatory bowel disease: a systematic review. Clin Gastroenterol Hepatol. 2014;12(9):1443–e89. https://doi.org/10.1016/j.cgh.2014.01.021.
19. Thaçi D, Papp K, Marcoux D, et al. Sustained long-term efficacy and safety of adalimumab in paediatric patients with severe chronic plaque psoriasis from a randomized, double-blind, phase III study. Br J Dermatol. 2019;181(6):1177–89. https://doi.org/10.1111/bjd.18029.
20. Bissonnette R, Bolduc C, Poulin Y, Guenther L, Lynde CW, Maari C. Efficacy and safety of adalimumab in patients with plaque psoriasis who have shown an unsatisfactory response to etanercept. J Am Acad Dermatol. 2010;63(2):228–34. https://doi.org/10.1016/j.jaad.2009.08.040.
21. Van Lümig PP, Lecluse LL, Driessen RJ, et al. Switching from etanercept to adalimumab is effective and safe: results in 30 patients with psoriasis with primary failure, secondary failure or intolerance to etanercept. Br J Dermatol. 2010;163(4):838–46. https://doi.org/10.1111/j.1365-2133.2010.09950.x.
22. Strober BE, Poulin Y, Kerdel FA, et al. Switching to adalimumab for psoriasis patients with a suboptimal response to etanercept, methotrexate, or phototherapy: efficacy and safety results from an open-label study. J Am Acad Dermatol. 2011;64(4):671–81. https://doi.org/10.1016/j.jaad.2010.03.009.
23. van der Heijde D, Deodhar A, FitzGerald O, et al. 4-year results from the RAPID-PsA phase 3 randomised placebo-controlled trial of certolizumab pegol in psoriatic arthritis published correction appears in RMD Open. 2018 Mar 26;4(1). RMD Open. 2018;4(1):e000582. Published 2018 Mar 14. https://doi.org/10.1136/rmdopen-2017-000582.
24. Atteno M, Peluso R, Costa L, et al. Comparison of effectiveness and safety of infliximab, etanercept, and adalimumab in psoriatic arthritis patients who experienced an inadequate response to previous disease-modifying antirheumatic drugs. 2010;29(4):399–403. https://doi.org/10.1007/s10067-009-1340-7.
25. Saad AA, Symmons DP, Noyce PR, Ashcroft DM. Risks and benefits of tumor necrosis factor-alpha inhibitors in the management of psoriatic arthritis: systematic review and metaanalysis of randomized controlled trials. J Rheumatol. 2008;35(5):883–90.
26. Fénix-Caballero S, Alegre-del Rey EJ, Castaño-Lara R, Puigventós-Latorre F, Borrero-Rubio JM, López-Vallejo JF. Direct and indirect comparison of the efficacy and safety of adalimumab, etanercept, infliximab and golimumab in psoriatic arthritis. J Clin Pharm Ther. 2013;38(4):286–93. https://doi.org/10.1111/jcpt.12045.
27. McInnes IB, Anderson JK, Magrey M, et al. Trial of Upadacitinib and adalimumab for psoriatic arthritis. N Engl J Med. 2021;384(13):1227–39. https://doi.org/10.1056/NEJMoa2022516.
28. Kavanaugh A, Husni ME, Harrison DD, et al. Safety and efficacy of intravenous Golimumab in patients with active psoriatic arthritis: results through week twenty-four of the GO-VIBRANT study. Arthritis Rheumatol. 2017;69(11):2151–61. https://doi.org/10.1002/art.40226.
29. Husni ME, Kavanaugh A, Murphy F, et al. Efficacy and safety of intravenous Golimumab through one year in patients with active psoriatic arthritis. Arthritis Care Res (Hoboken). 2020;72(6):806–13. https://doi.org/10.1002/acr.23905.
30. Kavanaugh A, McInnes I, Mease P, et al. Golimumab, a new human tumor necrosis factor alpha antibody, administered every four weeks as a subcutaneous injection in psoriatic arthritis: twenty-four-week efficacy and safety results of a randomized, placebo-controlled study [published correction appears in Arthritis Rheum.2010 Aug;62(8):2555]. Arthritis Rheum. 2009;60(4):976–86. https://doi.org/10.1002/art.2440.
31. Kavanaugh A, van der Heijde D, McInnes IB, et al. Golimumab in psoriatic arthritis: one-year clinical efficacy, radiographic, and safety results from a phase III, randomized, placebo-controlled trial. Arthritis Rheum. 2012;64(8):2504–17. https://doi.org/10.1002/art.3443.

32. The Lenercept Multiple Sclerosis Study Group and The University of British Columbia MS/MRI Analysis Group. TNF neutralization in MS: results of a randomized, placebo-controlled multicenter study. Neurology. 1999;53(3):457–65.
33. Garber C, Plotnikova N, Au SC, Sorensen EP, Gottlieb A. Biologic and conventional systemic therapies show similar safety and efficacy in elderly and adult patients with moderate to severe psoriasis. J Drugs Dermatol. 2015;14(8):846–52.
34. Strangfeld A, Eveslage M, Schneider M, et al. Treatment benefit or survival of the fittest: what drives the time-dependent decrease in serious infection rates under TNF inhibition and what does this imply for the individual patient? Ann Rheum Dis. 2011;70(11):1914–20. https://doi.org/10.1136/ard.2011.151043.
35. Singh JA, Wells GA, Christensen R, et al. Adverse effects of biologics: a network meta-analysis and Cochrane overview. Cochrane Database Syst Rev. 2011;2011(2):CD008794. Published 2011 Feb 16. https://doi.org/10.1002/14651858.CD008794.pub2.
36. Blauvelt A, et al. Long-term safety of certolizumab pegol in plaque psoriasis: pooled analysis over 3 years from three phase III, randomized, placebo-controlled studies. Br J Dermatol. 2021;184(4):640–51. https://doi.org/10.1111/bjd.19314.
37. Lau CS, et al. Tuberculosis and viral hepatitis in patients treated with certolizumab pegol in Asia-Pacific countries and worldwide: real-world and clinical trial data. Clin Rheumatol. 2021;40(3):867–75. https://doi.org/10.1007/s10067-020-05248-4.
38. Zhang Z, et al. Risk of tuberculosis in patients treated with TNF-α antagonists: a systematic review and meta-analysis of randomised controlled trials. BMJ open. 2017;7(3):e012567. https://doi.org/10.1136/bmjopen-2016-012567.
39. Daham N, AlMuqrin A, Madani A, AlSaif F. Fetal Acrania (Exencephaly) in the Context of a Pregnant Female Taking Adalimumab for Psoriasis: A Case Report. Biologics. 2020;14:127–9. Published 2020 Nov 11. https://doi.org/10.2147/BTT.S273762.
40. Bröms G, Kieler H, Ekbom A, et al. Anti-TNF treatment during pregnancy and birth outcomes: a population-based study from Denmark, Finland, and Sweden. Pharmacoepidemiol Drug Saf. 2020;29(3):316–27. https://doi.org/10.1002/pds.4930.
41. Owczarek W, Walecka I, Lesiak A, et al. The use of biological drugs in psoriasis patients prior to pregnancy, during pregnancy and lactation: a review of current clinical guidelines. Postepy Dermatol Alergol. 2020;37(6):821–30. https://doi.org/10.5114/ada.2020.102089.
42. Nielsen OH, Gubatan JM, Juhl CB, Streett SE, Maxwell C. Biologics for Inflammatory Bowel Disease and Their Safety in Pregnancy: A Systematic Review and Meta-analysis [published online ahead of print, 2020 Sep 12]. Clin Gastroenterol Hepatol. 2020;S1542–3565(20):31281–7. https://doi.org/10.1016/j.cgh.2020.09.021.
43. Hazlewood GS, Rezaie A, Borman M, et al. Comparative effectiveness of immunosuppressants and biologics for inducing and maintaining remission in Crohn's disease: a network meta-analysis. Gastroenterology. 2015;148(2):344–e15. https://doi.org/10.1053/j.gastro.2014.10.011.
44. Sandborn WJ, Feagan BG, Stoinov S, et al. Certolizumab pegol for the treatment of Crohn's disease. N Engl J Med. 2007;357(3):228–38. https://doi.org/10.1056/NEJMoa067594.
45. Sandborn WJ, Hanauer SB, Katz S, et al. Etanercept for active Crohn's disease: a randomized, double-blind, placebo-controlled trial. Gastroenterology. 2001;121(5):1088–94. https://doi.org/10.1053/gast.2001.28674.
46. Tubach F, Salmon D, Ravaud P, et al. Risk of tuberculosis is higher with anti-tumor necrosis factor monoclonal antibody therapy than with soluble tumor necrosis factor receptor therapy: the three-year prospective French Research Axed on Tolerance of Biotherapies registry [published correction appears in Arthritis Rheum. 2009 Aug;60(8):2540. Lortholary, O [corrected to Lortholary, O]]. Arthritis Rheum. 2009;60(7):1884–94. https://doi.org/10.1002/art.24632.
47. Pariser DM, Leonardi CL, Gordon K, et al. Integrated safety analysis: short- and long-term safety profiles of etanercept in patients with psoriasis. J Am Acad Dermatol. 2012;67(2):245–56. https://doi.org/10.1016/j.jaad.2011.07.040.
48. Gottlieb AB, Gordon K, Giannini EH, et al. Clinical trial safety and mortality analyses in patients receiving etanercept across approved indications. J Drugs Dermatol. 2011;10(3):289–300.
49. Lim JL, Stern RS. High levels of ultraviolet B exposure increase the risk of non-melanoma skin cancer in psoralen and ultraviolet A-treated patients. J Invest Dermatol. 2005;124(3):505–13. https://doi.org/10.1111/j.0022-202X.2005.23618.x.
50. Behnam SM, Behnam SE, Koo JY. Review of cyclosporine immunosuppressive safety data in dermatology patients after two decades of use. J Drugs Dermatol. 2005;4(2):189–94.
51. Margolis D, Bilker W, Hennessy S, Vittorio C, Santanna J, Strom BL. The risk of malignancy associated with psoriasis. Arch Dermatol. 2001;137(6):778–83.

4 IL-17 Class of Biologic Agents in Psoriatic Disease

Jennifer Soung, Samuel Stetkevich, and Momoko Ishizuka

Background Information IL-17

The IL-17 inflammatory pathway begins with dendritic cell activation that results in the release of interleukin-23 (IL-23). IL-23 then activates T helper 17 cells (Th17) resulting in the release of the IL-17 superfamily of cytokines which then bind to IL-17 receptor complexes. These receptor complexes are most abundantly expressed on hematopoietic cells but can also be found on epithelial cells, fibroblasts, keratinocytes, endothelial cells, monocytes, macrophages, and osteoblasts [1, 2]. The IL-17 cytokine superfamily consists of six members, IL-17A through IL-17F, and functions as a heterodimer IL-17A/F and homodimers IL-17A/A and IL-17F/F. IL-17A is the most potent receptor subtype in psoriasis, but IL-17F is the most prevalent. IL-17C also contributes to the release of pro-inflammatory cytokines during a psoriasis flare [3, 4]. IL-17E has mRNA expressions that are undetectable in psoriatic lesions. IL-17B and IL-17D are not well defined and do not play a significant role in the pathogenesis of psoriasis [5].

J. Soung (✉) · S. Stetkevich · M. Ishizuka
Southern California Dermatology, Inc., Santa Ana, CA, USA

Harbor University of California, Los Angeles, CA, USA
e-mail: JSoung@dhs.lacounty.gov

Secukinumab (Cosentyx)

Secukinumab (approved in 2015) is a fully human IgG1k monoclonal antibody that selectively binds and inhibits IL-17A. Secukinumab is approved for the treatment of moderate-to-severe plaque psoriasis, psoriatic arthritis, ankylosing spondylitis, and non-radiographic axial spondyloarthritis.

Phase III trials of secukinumab (ERASURE and FIXTURE) demonstrated effectiveness in the treatment of plaque psoriasis in 2044 adult patients with a PASI ≥12, BSA ≥ 10%, and IGA ≥ 3 [6, 7]. Key endpoints in these trials included the proportion of patients who achieved PASI 90 and PASI 100, an IGA 0 or 1 at week 12, and the mean score of Dermatology Life Quality Index (DLQI) with higher scores indicating a greater effect of the disease on quality of life [6, 7].

In both studies at week 12, a significantly greater proportion of patients on secukinumab achieved a PASI 90 compared to placebo or etanercept (in FIXTURE only): ERASURE, 300 mg 59.2%, placebo 1.2%; FIXTURE, 300 mg 54.2%, etanercept 20.7%, placebo 1.5%; $p < 0.001$ for all comparisons [6, 7]. PASI 100 results at week 12 yielded similar findings (ERASURE, 300 mg 28.6%, placebo 0.8%; FIXTURE, 300 mg 24.1%, etanercept 4.3%, placebo 0.0%; $p < 0.001$ for all comparisons) [6, 7]. Other comparative studies include secukinumab versus ustekinumab, an

N. Brownstone et al. (eds.), *Biologic Therapy for Psoriasis*, Updates in Clinical Dermatology,
https://doi.org/10.1007/978-3-030-92938-1_4

IL-12/IL-23 antagonist [CLEAR], and secukinumab versus guselkumab, an IL-23 antagonist [ECLIPSE]. Secukinumab demonstrated superiority to ustekinumab at week 16 with PASI 90 responses (CLEAR: secukinumab, 79.0%; ustekinumab, 57.6%; $p < 0.0001$) and PASI 100 responses (CLEAR: secukinumab, 44.3%; ustekinumab, 28.4%; $p < 0.0001$) [8]. Formal statistical testing of secukinumab versus guselkumab was not performed at week 16 with PASI 90 responses (ECLIPSE: secukinumab, 79.6%; guselkumab, 78.5%) and PASI 100 responses (ECLIPSE: secukinumab, 46.1%; guselkumab, 47.8%) [9]. However, guselkumab exhibited superiority to secukinumab at week 48 with PASI 90 responses (ECLIPSE: secukinumab, 70.0%; guselkumab, 84.5%; $p < 0.0001$) and PASI 100 responses (ECLIPSE: secukinumab, 48.4%; guselkumab, 58.2%; $p < 0.0001$) [9].

Similar results were produced in phase III studies of the pediatric population. The primary phase III study (NCT02471144) was a double-blind study assessing 162 patients aged 6 to <18 years with severe chronic plaque psoriasis [10]. The safety profile of secukinumab did not identify any new concerns with treatment of the pediatric population and demonstrated consistency with adult phase III studies [10].

In addition to the treatment of plaque psoriasis, secukinumab is also approved for the treatment of psoriatic arthritis. A phase III double-blind, placebo-controlled trial (FUTURE 2) demonstrated that a significantly higher proportion of patients achieved the primary endpoint of at least 20% improvement in the American College of Rheumatology response criteria (ACR20) at week 24 with secukinumab 300 mg (54% $p < 0.0001$), 150 mg (51% $p < 0.0001$), and 75 mg (29% $p = 0.0399$) versus placebo (15%) [11]. A more recent study further investigated how effectively secukinumab treats psoriatic arthritis. A parallel-group, double-blind, active-controlled, phase IIIb trial (EXCEED) compared secukinumab to adalimumab and proved the two medications have similar safety profiles and achieve similar ACR20 at week 52 (secukinumab, 67%; adalimumab, 62%; $p < 0.0719$) [12].

Secukinumab has also been studied for treatment of psoriasis in more challenging areas of the body such as the scalp and palmoplantar areas. Special site psoriasis treatment will be discussed later in Chap. 8.

Brodalumab (Siliq/Kyntheum)

Brodalumab, a human IgG2k monoclonal antibody, is unique among the IL-17 antagonists because it blocks IL-17A receptors, thus preventing IL-17A, IL-17F, IL-17A/F, and IL-17E activity. It is approved for the treatment of adult patients with moderate-to-severe plaque psoriasis who are candidates for systemic therapy or phototherapy *and* have failed to respond or have lost response to other systemic therapies.

Two phase III trials AMAGINE-2 and AMAGINE-3 were multicenter, randomized, double-blind, placebo-controlled and active comparator-controlled (ustekinumab), parallel-group, phase III trials which examined brodalumab vs. ustekinumab in adults [13]. Key endpoints of the trials included the proportion of patients who achieved PASI 90, PASI 100, and sPGA0 or 1 at week 12. The PASI 90 response at week 12 with brodalumab 210 mg was greater than ustekinumab and placebo (AMAGINE-2, 210 mg 70%, ustekinumab 47%, placebo 3%; AMAGINE-3, 210 mg 69%; ustekinumab 48%; placebo 2%; $p < 0.001$ for all comparisons) [7, 13]. The PASI 100 response rates at week 12 with brodalumab 210 mg were superior to ustekinumab and placebo (AMAGINE-2, 210 mg 44%, ustekinumab 22%, placebo 1%; AMAGINE-3, 210 mg 37%, ustekinumab 19%, placebo 0.3%; $p < 0.001$ for all comparisons) [7, 13]. The proportion of patients with sPGA of 0 or 1 at week 12 with 210 mg of brodalumab was greater than those with ustekinumab and placebo (AMAGINE-2, 210 mg 79%, ustekinumab 61%, placebo 4%; AMAGINE-3, 210 mg 80%, ustekinumab 57%, placebo 4%) [13]. The psoriasis symptom inventory (PSI) response achieved at week 12 with 210 mg of brodalumab was also superior to ustekinumab and placebo (AMAGINE-2, 210 mg 68%, ustekinumab 55%, placebo 7%; AMAGINE-3, 210 mg 61%, ustekinumab 52%, placebo 6%) [13].

Amgen and AstraZeneca halted the development program of brodalumab in May 2015 due to the emergence of a suicide signal. A total of six completed suicides in all brodalumab clinical trials were reported (four in psoriasis, one in rheumatoid arthritis, and one in psoriatic arthritis); however, one suicide was later adjudicated as indeterminate due to possible accidental drug overdose [14]. A recent pharmacovigilance report assessed the adverse effects of brodalumab and revealed no suicide attempts or completed suicides out of 2677 patients taking brodalumab [15]. Therefore, the original findings in the phase III trials with concerns to an increase in suicide risk appear to be inconclusive with the increase in data disproving this concern. Possible explanations for the original results might include underlying levels of depression and diminished quality of life experienced in patients with psoriasis.

Ixekizumab (Taltz)

Ixekizumab is approved for the treatment of patients ≥6 years or older with moderate-to-severe plaque psoriasis who are candidates for systemic therapy or phototherapy, adults with active psoriatic arthritis, adults with active ankylosing spondylitis (AS), and adults with active non-radiographic axial spondyloarthritis (nr-axSpA) with objective signs of inflammation. It is a recombinant, humanized IgG4-k monoclonal antibody that selectively binds and neutralizes IL-17A.

Safety and efficacy profiles of ixekizumab were evaluated in a series of phase III trials, UNCOVER-1, UNCOVER-2, and UNCOVER-3, in a total of 3866 adult psoriasis patients with BSA ≥ 10%, PASI score ≥ 12, and sPGA ≥3. At week 12, the PASI 90 response was significantly higher in patients treated with 80 mg ixekizumab Q2W than those with etanercept or placebo (UNCOVER-1, Q2W 70.9%, placebo 0.5%, $p < 0.001$; UNCOVER-2, Q2W 70.7%, etanercept 18.7%, placebo 0.6%, $p < 0.0001$; UNCOVER-3, Q2W 68.1%, etanercept 25.7%, placebo 3.1%, $p < 0.0001$) [16–18]. Patients with 80 mg ixekizumab Q2W also showed a greater PASI 100 response at week 12 compared to etanercept and placebo (UNCOVER-1, Q2W 35.3%, placebo 0.5%, $p < 0.001$; UNCOVER-2, Q2W 40.5%, etanercept 5.3%, placebo 0.6%, $p < 0.0001$; UNCOVER-3, Q2W 37.7%, etanercept 7.3%, placebo 0.0%, $p < 0.0001$) [16–18]. The proportion of patients with sPGA scores of 0/1 at week 12 was significantly higher with 80 mg ixekizumab Q2W (UNCOVER-1, Q2W 81.8%, placebo 3.2%, $p < 0.001$; UNCOVER-2, Q2W 83.2%, etanercept 36.0%, placebo 2.4%, $p < 0.0001$; UNCOVER-3, Q2W 80.5%, etanercept 41.6%, placebo 6.7%, $p < 0.0001$) [16–18].

In addition to plaque psoriasis, ixekizumab has been evaluated in difficult-to-treat areas including the scalp, nails, and palms and soles in the UNCOVER-1, UNCOVER-2, and UNCOVER-3 studies [19, 20]. To date, ixekizumab is the only biologic that has been evaluated for treatment of genital psoriasis with or without extensive plaque psoriasis [21]. At week 12, significantly more patients achieved a sPGA 0/1 of the genital area (73% versus placebo 8%, $p < 0.001$) [21]. Ixekizumab has also shown to be effective in treating patients with erythrodermic and generalized pustular psoriasis [22]. More details can be found in Chap. 8.

Several head-to-head studies comparing ixekizumab to other biologics have been reported. IXORA-S was the first head-to-head phase III trial evaluating the efficacy of ixekizumab versus ustekinumab. At week 12, 36.0% of patients with ixekizumab 80 mg Q2W achieved PASI 100 compared to 14.5% with ustekinumab, and 83.6% (ixekizumab Q2W) achieved sPGA 0/1 compared to 57.2% (ustekinumab) ($p < 0.001$) [23]. IXORA-R evaluated the efficacy of ixekizumab versus guselkumab. At week 12, 41% of patients with ixekizumab 80 mg Q2W achieved PASI 100 compared to 25% of patients with 100 mg guselkumab ($p < 0.001$) [24]. IXORA-PEDS was a phase III trial evaluating the safety and efficacy of ixekizumab in pediatric psoriasis patients ages 6 to <18 years. At week 12, 78% of patients with ixekizumab Q4W (weight-based dosing) achieved PASI 90 versus 5% placebo ($p < 0.001$) [25].

Ixekizumab is also approved for the treatment of active psoriatic arthritis. A phase III, double-blind trial (SPIRIT-P1) demonstrated that a significantly higher proportion of patients achieved at least an ACR20 when treated with ixekizumab Q2W (60.2%) and Q4W (57.0%) than placebo (31.1%, $p \leq 0.001$) and showed similar results to patients treated with adalimumab 40 mg (51.5%, $p \leq 0.01$) [26]. Another phase III, double-blind, placebo-controlled trial (SPIRIT-P2) investigated ixekizumab in 363 adult patients with active psoriatic arthritis who had a previous inadequate response to treatment with tumor necrosis factor (TNF) inhibitors. At week 24, a significantly higher proportion of patients achieved ACR20 when treated with ixekizumab Q2W (48%) and Q4W (53%) than placebo (19%, $p < 0.0001$) [27].

Bimekizumab (Bimzelx)

Bimekizumab is currently awaiting FDA approval for the treatment of adults with moderate-to-severe plaque psoriasis. Unlike secukinumab and ixekizumab, bimekizumab is a monoclonal IgGI antibody that selectively inhibits both IL-17A and IL-17F.

BE READY was a multicenter, double-blind, placebo-controlled phase III trial investigating the safety and efficacy of bimekizumab in adults. At week 16, 90.8% of patients on bimekizumab 320 mg Q4W achieved PASI 90, and 92.6% achieved IGA 0/1 compared to placebo (1.2% and 1.2%, respectively, $p < 0.0001$). PASI 100 was also significantly higher at week 16, 68.2% bimekizumab 320 mg Q4W vs 1.2% placebo ($p < 0.0001$) [28]. Bimekizumab demonstrated superiority to ustekinumab (BE VIVID) at week 16 with a PASI 90 response rate of 85% vs. 50% ustekinumab 45 or 95 mg and 5% placebo ($p < 0.0001$) [29]. In another head-to-head study comparing IL-17A/F inhibition (bimekizumab) versus only IL-17A (secukinumab), the PASI 90 response rate was significantly higher in patients treated with bimekizumab 320 mg Q4W than with secukinumab 300 mg Q4W (85.5% versus 74.3%, $p < 0.001$) [30].

BE ACTIVE was a phase II study evaluating bimekizumab for the treatment of adult patients with psoriatic arthritis. Bimekizumab was associated with significant improvements in ACR50 compared with placebo: 27% versus 41% versus 46% versus 24% versus 7%, respectively ($p = 0.0314$) [31]. Phase III studies of bimekizumab as a treatment for psoriatic arthritis are ongoing.

Drug Dosing and Side Effects

Each of the IL-17 medications is administered via a subcutaneous injection with unique dosing regimens. Please see table for dosing instructions (Table 4.1). The most common side effects among this class of medications include nasopharyngitis, upper respiratory infections, headaches, and *Candida* infections. Neutropenia also occurred more frequently than placebo [32]. Neutropenia levels were classified as mild and reversible not requiring laboratory monitoring. Because Th17 cells play a key role in mucocutaneous surveillance against extracellular pathogens, inhibition of IL-17A can result in increased *Candida* infections. *Candida* infections were more frequently observed in secukinumab (1.7%), ixekizumab (3.3%), brodalumab (4%), and bimekizumab (9.1%) [29, 33]. *Candida* infections were typically mild to moderate in severity, did not interrupt treatment, and resolved with appropriate therapy.

Because a small number of Crohn's disease and ulcerative colitis exacerbations or occurrences were observed in clinical trials for all IL-17 inhibitors, the risk of new onset or worsening of inflammatory bowel disease applies to all IL-17 antagonists, and brodalumab specifically states it is contraindicated in Crohn's disease. Brodalumab also carries a black box warning of a possible increased risk for suicidal ideation and behavior (SIB) [34]. Patients are required to enroll in the Risk Evaluation and Mitigation Strategy (REMS) program, which requires physicians to be certified to prescribe brodalumab,

Table 4.1 Anti-IL-17 agents and their properties

Drug	Brand name	Monoclonal antibody	Mechanism of action	Producing pharmaceutical organization	Dosage	Indication and phase
Secukinumab	Cosentyx	Fully human IgG1 anti-IL-17A	Neutralize IL-17A	Novartis	300 mg every week for five doses, then 300 mg SQ every month	FDA approved for PsO (2015) and PsA (2016); phase IV
Brodalumab	Siliq (USA), Kyntheum (Europe)	Fully human IgG2 anti-IL-17RA	Blocks receptor, inhibits IL-17A, IL-17A/F, IL-17F, IL-17E	Ortho dermatologics (USA) LEO Pharma (Europe)	210 mg every week for three doses, followed by 210 mg SQ every 2 weeks	FDA approved for PsO (2017): Phase IV
Ixekizumab	Taltz	Humanized IgG4 anti-IL-17A	Neutralize IL-17A	Eli Lilly	Initially 160 mg for one dose, followed by 80 mg after 2 weeks, then 80 mg every 2 weeks for five further doses (at weeks 4, 6, 8, 10 and 12), then 80 mg SQ every 4 weeks	FDA approved for PsO (2016) and PsA (2017); Phase IV
Bimekizumab	Bimzelx	Humanized IgG1 anti-IL-17A and anti-IL-17F	Neutralize IL-17A and IL-17F	UCB (Europe)	320mg Q4 week vs Q8 week Pending FDA approval	Pending FDA approval for PsO (Oct 2021); Phase III

PsO moderate-to-severe plaque psoriasis, *PsA* psoriatic arthritis, *SQ* subcutaneous injection, *URI* upper respiratory infection, *IBD* inflammatory bowel disease counsel patients on SIB, and report if patients discontinue therapy.

One other notable safety point among IL-17 antagonists is the lack of evidence of tuberculosis reactivation. An extensive literature review of 139 total articles, 23 of which met inclusion criteria, did not identify any cases of TB reactivation in patients treated with IL-17 inhibitors for psoriasis [35].

References

1. Hawkes JE, Yan BY, Chan TC, Krueger JG (2018) Discovery of the IL-23/IL-17 signaling pathway and the treatment of psoriasis. J Immunol. https://doi.org/10.4049/jimmunol.1800013
2. Wilson NJ, Boniface K, Chan JR, et al. (2007) Development, cytokine profile and function of human interleukin 17-producing helper T cells. Nat Immunol. https://doi.org/10.1038/ni1497
3. Fragoulis GE, Siebert S, Mcinnes IB (2016) Therapeutic targeting of IL-17 and IL-23 cytokines in immune-mediated diseases. Annu Rev Med. https://doi.org/10.1146/annurev-med-051914-021944.
4. Ly K, Smith MP, Thibodeaux Q, Reddy V, Liao W, Bhutani T (2019) Anti IL-17 in psoriasis. Expert Rev Clin Immunol. https://doi.org/10.1080/1744666X.2020.1679625.
5. Yamauchi PS, Bagel J (2015) Next-generation biologics in the management of plaque psoriasis: a literature review of IL-17 inhibition. Journal of drugs in Dermatology. 14.
6. Langley RG, Elewski BE, Lebwohl M, et al. (2014) Secukinumab in plaque psoriasis — results of two phase 3 trials. N Engl J Med. https://doi.org/10.1056/nejmoa1314258.
7. Menter A, Strober BE, Kaplan DH, et al. (2019) Joint AAD-NPF guidelines of care for the management and treatment of psoriasis with biologics. J Am Acad Dermatol. https://doi.org/10.1016/j.jaad.2018.11.057.
8. Thaçi D, Blauvelt A, Reich K, et al. (2015) Secukinumab is superior to ustekinumab in clearing skin of subjects with moderate to severe plaque psoriasis: CLEAR, a randomized controlled trial. J Am Acad Dermatol. https://doi.org/10.1016/j.jaad.2015.05.013.
9. Reich K, Armstrong AW, Langley RG, Flavin S, Randazzo B, Li S, Hsu MC, Branigan P, Blauvelt A (2019) Guselkumab versus secukinumab for the treatment of moderate-to-severe psoriasis (ECLIPSE): results from a phase 3, randomised controlled trial. Lancet. https://doi.org/10.1016/S0140-6736(19)31773-8.
10. Bodemer C, Kaszuba A, Kingo K, et al. (2021) Secukinumab demonstrates high efficacy and a favourable safety profile in paediatric patients with severe chronic plaque psoriasis: 52-week results from a phase 3 double-blind randomized, controlled trial. J Eur Acad Dermatol Venereol. https://doi.org/10.1111/jdv.17002.
11. McInnes IB, Mease PJ, Kirkham B, et al. (2015) Secukinumab, a human anti-interleukin-17A monoclonal antibody, in patients with psoriatic arthritis (FUTURE 2): a randomised, double-blind, placebo-controlled, phase 3 trial. Lancet. https://doi.org/10.1016/S0140-6736(15)61134-5.
12. McInnes IB, Behrens F, Mease PJ, et al. (2020) Secukinumab versus adalimumab for treatment of active psoriatic arthritis (EXCEED): a double-blind, parallel-group, randomised, active-controlled, phase 3b trial. Lancet (London, England). https://doi.org/10.1016/S0140-6736(20)30564-X.
13. Lebwohl M, Strober B, Menter A, et al. Phase 3 studies comparing Brodalumab with Ustekinumab in psoriasis. N Engl J Med. 2015; https://doi.org/10.1056/nejmoa1503824.
14. Foulkes AC, Warren RB (2019) Brodalumab in psoriasis: evidence to date and clinical potential. Drugs Context. https://doi.org/10.7573/dic.212570.
15. Lebwohl M, Leonardi C, Wu JJ, Armstrong A, Rawnsley N, Merchant M, Alexander B, Jacobson A. Two-year US pharmacovigilance report on Brodalumab. Dermatol Ther. 2021; https://doi.org/10.1007/s13555-020-00472-x.
16. Gordon KB, Blauvelt A, Papp KA, et al. (2016) Phase 3 trials of Ixekizumab in moderate-to-severe plaque psoriasis. N Engl J Med. https://doi.org/10.1056/nejmoa1512711.
17. Papp KA, Leonardi CL, Blauvelt A, et al. Ixekizumab treatment for psoriasis: integrated efficacy analysis of three double-blinded, controlled studies (UNCOVER-1, UNCOVER-2, UNCOVER-3). Br J Dermatol. 2018; https://doi.org/10.1111/bjd.16050.
18. Griffiths CEM, Reich K, Lebwohl M, et al. Comparison of ixekizumab with etanercept or placebo in moderate-to-severe psoriasis (UNCOVER-2 and UNCOVER-3): results from two phase 3 randomised trials. Lancet. 2015; https://doi.org/10.1016/S0140-6736(15)60125-8.
19. Reich K, Leonardi C, Lebwohl M, Kerdel F, Okubo Y, Romiti R, Goldblum O, Dennehy EB, Kerr L, Sofen H (2017) Sustained response with ixekizumab treatment of moderate-to-severe psoriasis with scalp involvement: results from three phase 3 trials (UNCOVER-1, UNCOVER-2, UNCOVER-3). J Dermatol Treat. https://doi.org/10.1080/09546634.2016.1249820.
20. Menter A, Warren RB, Langley RG, Merola JF, Kerr LN, Dennehy EB, Shrom D, Amato D, Okubo Y, Reich K (2017) Efficacy of ixekizumab compared to etanercept and placebo in patients with moderate-to-severe plaque psoriasis and non-pustular palmoplantar involvement: results from three phase 3 trials (UNCOVER-1, UNCOVER-2 and UNCOVER-3). J

Eur Acad Dermatol Venereol. https://doi.org/10.1111/jdv.14237.
21. Ryan C, Menter A, Guenther L, et al. (2018) Efficacy and safety of ixekizumab in a randomized, double-blinded, placebo-controlled phase IIIb study of patients with moderate-to-severe genital psoriasis. Br J Dermatol. https://doi.org/10.1111/bjd.16736.
22. Saeki H, Nakagawa H, Nakajo K, et al. (2017) Efficacy and safety of ixekizumab treatment for Japanese patients with moderate to severe plaque psoriasis, erythrodermic psoriasis and generalized pustular psoriasis: results from a 52-week, open-label, phase 3 study (UNCOVER-J). J Dermatol. https://doi.org/10.1111/1346-8138.13622.
23. Reich K, Pinter A, Lacour JP, et al. (2017) Comparison of ixekizumab with ustekinumab in moderate-to-severe psoriasis: 24-week results from IXORA-S, a phase III study. Br J Dermatol. https://doi.org/10.1111/bjd.15666.
24. Blauvelt A, Papp K, Gottlieb A, et al. A head-to-head comparison of ixekizumab vs. guselkumab in patients with moderate-to-severe plaque psoriasis: 12-week efficacy, safety and speed of response from a randomized, double-blinded trial. Br J Dermatol. 2020; https://doi.org/10.1111/bjd.18851.
25. Paller AS, Seyger MMB, Alejandro Magariños G, et al. Efficacy and safety of ixekizumab in a phase III, randomized, double-blind, placebo-controlled study in paediatric patients with moderate-to-severe plaque psoriasis (IXORA-PEDS). Br J Dermatol. 2020; https://doi.org/10.1111/bjd.19147.
26. Mease PJ, van der Heijde D, Ritchlin CT, Okada M, Cuchacovich RS, Shuler CL, Lin CY, Braun DK, Lee CH, Gladman DD. Ixekizumab, an interleukin-17A specific monoclonal antibody, for the treatment of biologic-naive patients with active psoriatic arthritis: results from the 24-week randomised, double-blind, placebo-controlled and active (adalimumab)-controlled period of the phase III trial SPIRIT-P1. Ann Rheum Dis. 2017; https://doi.org/10.1136/annrheumdis-2016-209709.
27. Nash P, Kirkham B, Okada M, et al. Ixekizumab for the treatment of patients with active psoriatic arthritis and an inadequate response to tumour necrosis factor inhibitors: results from the 24-week randomised, double-blind, placebo-controlled period of the SPIRIT-P2 phase 3 trial. Lancet. 2017; https://doi.org/10.1016/S0140-6736(17)31429-0.
28. Gordon KB, Foley P, Krueger JG, et al. (2021) Bimekizumab efficacy and safety in moderate to severe plaque psoriasis (BE READY): a multicentre, double-blind, placebo-controlled, randomised withdrawal phase 3 trial. Lancet. https://doi.org/10.1016/S0140-6736(21)00126-4.
29. Reich K, Papp KA, Blauvelt A, et al. Bimekizumab versus ustekinumab for the treatment of moderate to severe plaque psoriasis (BE VIVID): efficacy and safety from a 52-week, multicentre, double-blind, active comparator and placebo controlled phase 3 trial. Lancet. 2021; https://doi.org/10.1016/S0140-6736(21)00125-2.
30. Reich K, Warren RB, Lebwohl M, et al. Bimekizumab versus Secukinumab in Plaque Psoriasis. N Engl J Med. 2021; https://doi.org/10.1056/nejmoa2102383.
31. Ritchlin CT, Kavanaugh A, Merola JF, et al. Bimekizumab in patients with active psoriatic arthritis: results from a 48-week, randomised, double-blind, placebo-controlled, dose-ranging phase 2b trial. Lancet. 2020; https://doi.org/10.1016/S0140-6736(19)33161-7.
32. Silfvast-Kaiser A, Paek SY, Menter A. Anti-IL17 therapies for psoriasis. Expert Opin Biol Ther. 2019; https://doi.org/10.1080/14712598.2019.1555235.
33. Saunte DM, Mrowietz U, Puig L, Zachariae C. Candida infections in patients with psoriasis and psoriatic arthritis treated with interleukin-17 inhibitors and their practical management. Br J Dermatol. 2017; https://doi.org/10.1111/bjd.15015.
34. Lebwohl MG, Papp KA, Marangell LB, et al. Psychiatric adverse events during treatment with brodalumab: analysis of psoriasis clinical trials. J Am Acad Dermatol. 2018; https://doi.org/10.1016/j.jaad.2017.08.024.
35. Fowler E, Ghamrawi RI, Ghiam N, Liao W, Wu JJ (2020) Risk of tuberculosis reactivation during interleukin-17 inhibitor therapy for psoriasis: a systematic review. J Eur Acad Dermatol Venereol. https://doi.org/10.1111/jdv.16254.

IL-23 Class of Biologic Agents in Psoriatic Disease

5

Jason E. Hawkes

Introduction

Psoriasis vulgaris is a common, heterogeneous, chronic inflammatory disease typified by raised, red, plaques with a prominent white scale that is frequently found on the extensor surfaces of the extremities, trunk, scalp, and acral skin. While the exact etiology of psoriatic disease is unknown, the condition is characterized by systemic inflammation, a central T cell-mediated immune response, and an increased risk for developing other psoriasis-associated conditions or comorbidities [1]. Known comorbidities of psoriasis include cardiovascular disease, stroke, hypertension, diabetes, obesity and metabolic syndrome, inflammatory arthritis, chronic kidney disease, inflammatory bowel disease, sleep disorders, and psychosocial stress/mood disorders [2].

The lifelong impact that psoriasis has on the estimated 3% of the USA affected by this disease is tremendous and represents a large economic burden on our healthcare infrastructure [3]. The ability to access long-term, clinically effective, durable, and safe systemic treatments by psoriasis patients and healthcare providers is essential. The elucidation of the IL-23/17 signaling pathway and its central role in the development of psoriasis is arguably the single most important discovery to date in psoriatic disease research due to the sheer number and success of systemic treatments that were developed as a result of its discovery [4]. Targeted blockade of IL-23 signaling via IL-12/23 (ustekinumab) and IL-23 (guselkumab, tildrakizumab, risankizumab) has set a new clinical standard for disease improvement, treatment durability, and overall safety in psoriatic disease. This chapter will focus on the discovery of the IL-23 signaling pathway and its role in the immunopathogenesis of psoriasis, as well as the pharmacologic and safety profiles observed with biologics in this treatment class (Table 5.1) for plaque psoriasis and psoriatic arthritis.

A History of Psoriatic Disease and the Discovery of the Central IL-23/17 Signaling Axis

Following early laboratory and clinical observations in the late twentieth century suggesting that psoriasis was inextricably linked to an activated immune response, efforts began to repurpose and investigate existing immunotherapies for the treatment of plaque psoriasis. These early observations included the clinical resolution of plaque psoriasis in cancer patients undergoing chemotherapy, bone marrow and organ transplant

J. E. Hawkes (✉)
Department of Dermatology, University of California-Davis, Sacramento, CA, USA
e-mail: jehawkes@ucdavis.edu

N. Brownstone et al. (eds.), *Biologic Therapy for Psoriasis*, Updates in Clinical Dermatology,
https://doi.org/10.1007/978-3-030-92938-1_5

Table 5.1 Overview of FDA-approved biologics that inhibit IL-23

Name (brand)	Manufacturer	Target	Approved indication (year)	Subcutaneous dosing schedule
Ustekinumab (Stelara)	Janssen	IL-12, IL-23 (p40 subunit)	Ps (2009) PsA (2013)	*Adults (18 and older)* <100 kg = 45 mg at weeks 0 and 4, then every 12 weeks >100 kg = 90 mg at weeks 0 and 4, then every 12 weeks. *Children (6–17 years)* <60 kg = 0.75 mg/kg at weeks 0 and 4, then every 12 weeks 60–100 kg = 45 mg at weeks 0 and 4, then every 12 weeks >100 kg = 90 mg at weeks 0 and 4, then every 12 weeks
Guselkumab (Tremfya)	Janssen	IL-23 (p19 subunit)	Ps (2017) PsA (2020)	100 mg given at weeks 0 and 4, then every 8 weeks
Tildrakizumab (Ilumya)	Sun Pharma	IL-23 (p19 subunit)	Ps (2018)	100 mg given at weeks 0 and 4, then every 12 weeks with administration given by a healthcare provider
Risankizumab (Skyrizi)	AbbVie	IL-23 (p19 subunit)	Ps (2019)	150 mg given at weeks 0 and 4, then every 12 weeks.

Abbreviations: *Ps* plaque psoriasis, *PsA* psoriatic arthritis

recipients requiring ongoing immunosuppression, and the identification of $CD4^+$ and $CD8^+$ T cell infiltrates in the lesional skin of patients with psoriatic disease [5–8]. As a result, there were several decades where psoriatic disease was primarily treated with systemic immunosuppressants (e.g., methotrexate and cyclosporine), modulators of keratinocyte differentiation (e.g., acitretin), or light-based treatments (e.g., Goeckerman therapy and narrowband UVB). The broad-acting, nonspecific mechanism of these oral systemic therapies and their narrow therapeutic index limited their use in many patients and/or were contraindicated due to other concomitant medications and preexisting medical conditions (e.g., kidney disease and pregnancy). Light-based therapies, on the other hand, required the expertise and proper equipment to perform such treatments and were inconvenient and costly (e.g., co-payment associated with each treatment session) for many patients. There was a clear need for additional treatment modalities.

Selective inhibition of activated T lymphocytes in psoriasis patients via a novel fusion protein composed of human IL-2 and diphtheria toxin fragments (DAB389IL-2) provided definitive proof for the link between T cells and plaque psoriasis [9]. Novel proof-of-concept studies showing the clinical effectiveness of targeted immunotherapies such as abatacept (fusion protein of the Fc region of the immunoglobulin IgG1 and the extracellular domain of CTLA-4) [10], alefacept (CD2-directed LFA-3/Fc fusion protein) [11], and efalizumab (a recombinant humanized monoclonal antibody against CD11a) [12] further underscored the central role of the T lymphocyte in the development of psoriasis and paved the way for the prospect of developing targeted therapies against other immune cells or their pro-inflammatory proteins. Targeted immunotherapies offered promise by having the potential benefit of interrupting the dysregulated immune response driving psoriatic disease, while lacking the untoward adverse effects associated with broad-acting systemic immunosuppressants like methotrexate, cyclosporine, or acitretin. The first report of a patient with refractory Crohn's disease and widespread plaque psoriasis successfully treated for both conditions using an intravenous humanized anti-TNFα monoclonal antibody (i.e., infliximab) irrevocably changed the therapeutic landscape in dermatology and firmly established biologics as an advantageous treatment class over traditional systemic immunosuppressants for most patients with widespread disease [13]. Additional reports of the successful treatment of moderate-to-severe plaque psoriasis via subcutaneously administered monoclonal antibodies against TNFα and the ensuing FDA approval of etanercept (2003) and adalimumab (2008) were key milestones that further expanded the armamentarium of available therapeutic options for plaque psoriasis and improved treatment access for a significant number of affected patients.

As anti-TNFα agents took center stage for the treatment of psoriasis and other inflammatory conditions, ongoing research and "gene hunting" efforts were searching to identify other potential markers of chronic inflammatory and autoimmune diseases [14]. The prevailing hypothesis at the time was that autoimmune disease was primarily driven by the Th1 subset and its primary regulatory cytokine, IL-12, a heterodimeric protein composed of the p35 and p40 subunits. These research efforts led to the prediction and subsequent identification of multiple heterodimeric cytokines that were structurally similar to IL-12 (e.g., IL-23 and IL-39), thus expanding the IL-12 cytokine family [14]. Pairing of a novel p19 subunit combined with the p40 subunit resulted in a novel cytokine later named IL-23, whereas the pairing of the p19 and EBI3 subunits resulted in the IL-39 cytokine (Fig. 5.1). IL-23 is produced by activated phagocytic and dendritic cell populations and is a key signal in the cutaneous protection against bacterial, viral, and fungal pathogens [15]. The function of IL-39 has not been clearly established and does not appear to play a role in the etiology of psoriasis.

Studies aimed at determining whether IL-23, like IL-12, might regulate autoimmune disease and the Th1 subset ultimately found that IL-23 regulated a subset of IL-17-producing $CD4^+$ T lymphocytes that were negative for traditional Th1 and Th2 markers. This challenged the prevailing, conventional Th1/Th2 classification that was common at that time [16]. Landmark murine

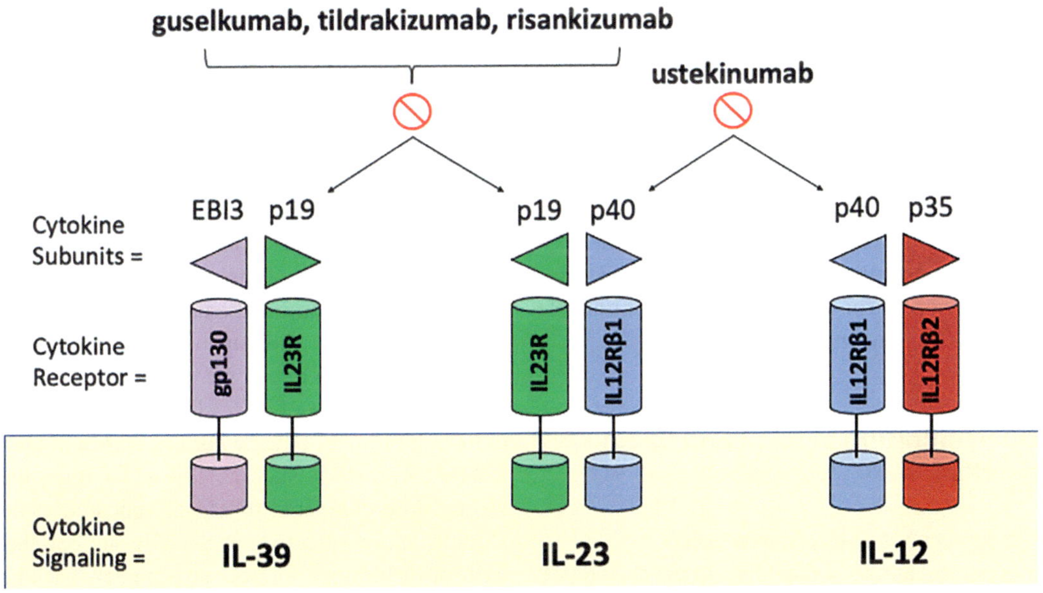

Fig. 5.1 Schematic showing the specific cytokine subunits and associated cell surface receptors involved in the signaling of IL-39, IL-23, and IL-12, as well as the mechanism of action for current FDA-approved biologics that selectively inhibit IL-23 via p19 (guselkumab, tildrakizumab, risankizumab) or dual inhibition of IL-12/23 via p40 (ustekinumab)

experiments and subsequent investigations provided definitive proof of an IL-17-producing T helper (Th17) population that was under the regulatory control of IL-23 and mediated an inflammatory phenotype in mice that could be neutralized by p40 (i.e., IL-12 and IL-23) or p19 inhibition (i.e., IL-23 with no impact on IL-12) but showed disease worsening with p35 inhibition (i.e., IL-12 alone with no impact on IL-23) [17, 18]. Worsening of the autoinflammatory phenotype in mice with IL-12p35 inhibition suggested a potentially protective role for IL-12 in certain inflammatory conditions and argued that IL-23, rather than IL-12, was the primary cytokine responsible for prior disease improvements seen with p40 subunit inhibition. Lesional skin from psoriatic plaques were later shown to have elevated numbers of IL-17-producing lymphocytes [19, 20] as well as the p40 and p19 subunits [21] with no increase in p35, therefore reinforcing the finding that IL-23 was the primary regulator of IL-17-producing cells. Efforts to directly block IL-17 and/or the expansion of Th17 cells via IL-23p19 inhibition in patients with plaque psoriasis suddenly took hold and provided hope for psoriasis patients who had not responded adequately to TNFα blockade. Working models for psoriatic disease were later updated to incorporate IL-23 and Th17 cells as the primary signaling axis in plaque psoriasis [22]. Novel biologic therapies that block both IL-12 and IL-23 via inhibition of the p40 subunit (ustekinumab) or selective inhibition of IL-23 alone via the p19 subunit (guselkumab, tildrakizumab, risankizumab) along with their successful phase 3 clinical trials lend strong support for the central role of IL-23/17 signaling in psoriasis.

Dual Inhibition of IL-12 and IL-23: Ustekinumab

Ustekinumab is a fully human IgG1κ monoclonal antibody that binds to the shared p40 subunit of the IL-12 and IL-23 cytokines as outlined above and in Fig. 5.1. Ustekinumab, therefore, inhibits both the Th1 and Th17 cell populations in psoriatic disease via a reduction of the two cytokines (IL-12 and IL-23) that drive the stimulation and expansion of these specific T helper subsets, respectively. The efficacy and safety of ustekinumab were established by three major phase 3 clinical trials: PHOENIX I and II [23, 24] as well as a head-to-head study with etanercept [25]. Following these trials, ustekinumab received FDA approval for moderate-to-severe plaque psoriasis in 2009; FDA approval for ustekinumab for the treatment of psoriatic arthritis was announced in 2013. It is administered subcutaneously as a 45 mg (<100 kg patient body weight) or 90 mg (>100 kg) injection on weeks 0 and 4 and then every 12 weeks (3 months) for plaque psoriasis and psoriatic arthritis, though some patients may require it every 8 weeks to maintain symptom control. Ustekinumab is also approved for the treatment of moderate-to-severe plaque psoriasis in children aged 6 or older based on weight: <60 kg = 0.75 mg/kg subcutaneous injection on weeks 0 and 4 and then every 12 weeks, 60–100 kg = 45 mg subcutaneous injection on weeks 0 and 4 and then every 12 weeks, and > 100 kg = 90 mg subcutaneous injection on weeks 0 and 4 and then every 12 weeks.

The clinical efficacy of ustekinumab in the PHOENIX I and II trials for plaque psoriasis showed 75% improvement in the psoriasis area and severity index score (PASI 75) in approximately 67% and 85% of patients at week 12 (45 mg dose) and week 24 (90 mg dose), respectively [23, 24]. Most patients had a durable clinical response after discontinuation of treatment (i.e., no rapid return of disease in the absence of treatment) with some patients staying clear for more than 1 year without the need for further treatment; this was one of the first clues revealing the dramatic effect of IL-23 blockade compared to the inhibition of other cytokines known to contribute to psoriasis such as TNFα. Of note, the 90 mg dose compared to 45 mg appeared to be slightly more effective, especially in patients with prior biologic failures or a higher baseline body weight. Seventy percent of ustekinumab-treated patients achieved a PASI 75 response compared to only 57% of those receiving etanercept as part of the head-to-head ACCEPT trial

[25]. Phase 3 trials also established ustekinumab as a durable therapeutic option with more than 80% of PASI 75 responders maintaining their clinical response through 5 years [26]. Very similar PASI 75 results were observed in pediatric patients with plaque psoriasis treated with ustekinumab [27].

Ustekinumab has also been studied and shown to be effective for the treatment of psoriatic arthritis in the PSUMMIT 1 and 2 trials [28, 29]. In the PSUMMIT trials, 42–50% of patients achieved 20% improvement in the American College of Rheumatology disease activity core measures (ACR 20) after 24 weeks with the highest symptom improvements seen in those receiving the 90 mg dose. Patients also noted improvement in dactylitis and enthesitis symptoms further supporting the efficacy of ustekinumab in psoriatic arthritis. The improvement in joint symptoms during the PSUMMIT trials was also maintained in patients through 52 weeks.

In general, the 90 mg dose of ustekinumab is preferred in patients with both plaque psoriasis and psoriatic arthritis given every 12 weeks or every 8 weeks for those with refractory disease or inadequately controlled symptoms. Though ustekinumab received FDA approval for psoriatic arthritis in 2013, its efficacy for psoriatic arthritis is generally felt to be lower than that of most TNFα inhibitors. Whether the lack of superiority of ustekinumab for the treatment of psoriatic arthritis is related to its inhibition and loss of the protective effects of IL-12 is unclear, although it is an interesting hypothesis given the apparent superiority of selective IL-23p19 antagonists for psoriatic arthritis compared to TNFα inhibitors (discussed below).

Selective Blockade of IL-23: Guselkumab, Tildrakizumab, and Risankizumab

In contrast to ustekinumab, which inhibits both IL-12 and IL-23, selective inhibitors of the p19 subunit leverage the advantages of IL-23 blockade for the treatment of plaque psoriasis while persevering the potentially beneficial effects of IL-12 (i.e., reduced psoriasiform dermatitis and infiltration of IL-17-producing cells into the skin) [30]. There are currently three selective IL-23 inhibitors approved in the USA for the treatment of psoriatic disease: guselkumab, tildrakizumab, and risankizumab.

Guselkumab

Guselkumab is a fully human IgG1λ monoclonal antibody that binds the p19 subunit of IL-23 as outlined above and illustrated in Fig. 5.1. The efficacy and safety of guselkumab for the treatment of moderate-to-severe plaque psoriasis were established by three major phase 3 studies: the VOYAGE 1 and 2 [31, 32] and NAVIGATE [33] trials. Another phase 3 study (ECLIPSE) [34] compared the efficacy of guselkumab to secukinumab, the first direct comparator study of a selective IL-23p19 inhibitor versus an IL-17A antagonist. Guselkumab received FDA approval for the treatment of plaque psoriasis in 2017, followed by an approval for psoriatic arthritis in 2020. It is administered as a 100 mg subcutaneous injection given at weeks 0 and 4 and then every 8 weeks. Guselkumab is the only IL-23 antagonist currently approved for the treatment of both moderate-to-severe plaque psoriasis and psoriatic arthritis.

The Phase 3 VOYAGE trials showed that 86–91% and 70–73% of plaque psoriasis patients achieved a PASI 75 and PASI 90, respectively, at week 16 compared to only about 70% of patients treated with adalimumab [31, 32]. Importantly, PASI 90 scores continued to improve beyond week 16 through week 24 with most patients maintaining high skin clearance rates through all study endpoints. As observed with ustekinumab, the VOYAGE studies for guselkumab also demonstrated a strong inhibition of skin disease following treatment cessation. Nevertheless, overall IL-23 suppression appears to be more complete in patients receiving guselkumab compared to ustekinumab since patients with inadequate treatment responses to ustekinumab improved with guselkumab rescue as shown in the NAVIGATE phase 3 trial [33]. The precise reason behind treatment response differences observed with IL-12/23p40 (ustekinumab) versus IL-23p19 (e.g., guselkumab) blockade is not completely understood and is currently being investigated. Finally, in the landmark ECLIPSE study [34] evaluating the relative efficacy of guselkumab versus secukinumab (anti-IL-17A monoclonal antibody), secukinumab appeared to have a slightly faster onset of action at early study endpoints though guselkumab performed similarly mid-study and slightly better at week 48 with a greater proportion of patients achieving and maintaining PASI 90. Two IXORA-R phase 4 studies that were similar in design to the ECLIPSE study compared guselkumab versus ixekizumab for the treatment of plaque psoriasis and revealed a similar efficacy (i.e., PASI 100) at week 24 [35, 36].

Guselkumab has also been shown to be effective for the treatment of psoriatic arthritis as demonstrated in two pivotal phase 3 trials: DISCOVER-1 and DISCOVER-2 [37, 38]. Both studies showed significant improvement in psoriatic arthritis symptoms compared to placebo with guselkumab achieving ACR 20 in approximately 60% of patients by week 24. Q4 week dosing of guselkumab for psoriatic arthritis versus Q8 week dosing did not appear to be consistently better for joint symptoms. The efficacy of other IL-23 antagonists (e.g., tildrakizumab and risankizumab) for the treatment of psoriatic arthritis has not yet been fully established, though the likelihood that they will receive FDA approval for this indication is considered highly likely given the success observed with guselkumab.

Tildrakizumab

Tildrakizumab is a fully human IgG1κ monoclonal antibody that also binds the p19 subunit of IL-23. The efficacy and safety of tildrakizumab were established by two pivotal phase 3 trials: reSURFACE 1 and 2 [39]. Tildrakizumab received FDA approval for the treatment of moderate-to-severe plaque psoriasis in 2018. Unlike guselkumab and risankizumab, tildrakizumab much be administered by a healthcare provider. It is administered as a single 100 mg subcutaneous injection at weeks 0 and 4 and then every 12 weeks. Tildrakizumab is not currently approved for the treatment of psoriatic arthritis.

In the reSURFACE studies, two-thirds of patients achieved PASI 75 at week 12 for the 100 mg and 200 mg treatment arms and were superior to etanercept [39]. Approximately one-third of patients achieved a PASI 100 at the same week 12 endpoint. A cursory review of the week 12 data for tildrakizumab compared to guselkumab and risankizumab might lead one to conclude that tildrakizumab is an inferior IL-23 antagonist. Rather, the PASI scores for tildrakizumab continue to improve significantly beyond week 12 through week 28 with a near doubling of the PASI 100 percentage suggesting a slower onset or delayed clinical response that requires a longer treatment period before maximal efficacy is achieved in plaque psoriasis patients. The clinical response associated with tildrakizumab is also sustained in most patients through 5 years with no safety signals beyond the adverse event profile discussed below [40]. Tildrakizumab is also an excellent cost-effective treatment compared to other biologics and small molecules such as apremilast [41].

Phase 2 clinical trials for tildrakizumab for the treatment of psoriatic arthritis are complete, while phase 3 studies are currently ongoing (NCT04314544, NCT04314531, NCT04991116). Careful evaluation of the future phase 3 data will be helpful to determine the relative efficacy of tildrakizumab versus guselkumab and TNFα inhibitors for the treatment of psoriatic arthritis and may expand the treatment options we have for this clinical variant.

Risankizumab

Risankizumab is a fully human IgG1 monoclonal antibody that also binds the p19 subunit of IL-23. The efficacy and safety of risankizumab were established by two pivotal phase 3 trials: UltIMMa-1 and UltIMMa-2 [42]. Risankizumab received FDA approval for the treatment of moderate-to-severe plaque psoriasis in 2019. It is administered as two 75 mg (150 mg) subcutaneous injections at weeks 0 and 4 and then every 12 weeks. Risankizumab is not currently approved for the treatment of psoriatic arthritis.

In the UltIMMa studies, risankizumab was associated with a PASI 90 in approximately 75% of patients at week 16 with as many as 80% achieving PASI 90 by week 52 [42]. Compared to other IL-23 inhibitors (i.e., guselkumab and tildrakizumab), risankizumab appears to be associated with a higher percentage of patients achieving PASI 90 and PASI 100 at the same week 16 timepoint. This higher rate of skin clearance with risankizumab is also observed in comparative trials with other biologic agents including adalimumab (IMMvent study) [43], ustekinumab [44], and secukinumab (IMMerge study) [45]. The IMMerge study comparing risankizumab and secukinumab for the treatment of plaque psoriasis is of particular interest given the prior guselkumab versus secukinumab (ECLIPSE) and guselkumab versus ixekizumab (IXORA-R) trials. Results from the IMMerge study revealed a comparable efficacy for risankizumab and secukinumab in the first 8 weeks of the study but clear divergence between the two biologics at week 16 with statistical superiority for risankizumab at week 20 through week 52 [45]. While further head-to-head trials comparing the treatment differences between IL-23 and IL-17 antagonists for psoriatic disease are interesting, they are unlikely to provide additional clinical information that would significantly impact current clinical decision-making given the high efficacy of both biologic classes for the treatment of skin disease.

Phase 2 clinical trials for risankizumab for the treatment of psoriatic arthritis are complete, while phase 3 studies are currently ongoing (NCT03675308, NCT03671148). Early phase 3 study data from the KEEPsAKE 1 (NCT03675308) and 2 (NCT03671148) trials suggests a positive effect of risankizumab on psoriatic joint disease symptoms and would compete with guselkumab as a potential first-line agent for the treatment of psoriatic arthritis. Careful evaluation of the future phase 3 data will be helpful to determine the relative efficacy of risankizumab versus guselkumab and TNFα inhibitors for the treatment of psoriatic arthritis and may expand the treatment options we have for this clinical variant.

Mirikizumab

Mirikizumab is a humanized monoclonal IgG4 variant antibody that also blocks the p19 subunit of IL-23. Despite good efficacy and safety for the treatment of moderate-to-severe plaque psoriasis observed in phase 3 clinical trials, OASIS-1 (NCT03482011) and OASIS-2 (NCT03535194), Eli Lilly and Company made the decision to not pursue regulatory approval for mirikizumab in plaque psoriasis possibly due to a crowded treatment class for this condition. Instead, the company is pursuing approval for mirikizumab in other indications such as the treatment of ulcerative colitis and Crohn's disease. Given the focus on psoriatic disease in this chapter, the clinical trial data for this antibody in other inflammatory conditions will not be reviewed here.

Safety Profiles of Ustekinumab, Guselkumab, Tildrakizumab, and Risankizumab

The safety profiles for ustekinumab, as well as guselkumab, tildrakizumab, and risankizumab, are excellent and arguably the safest biologics when compared to TNFα and IL-17 antagonists. The most common adverse events for ustekinumab include headache, upper respiratory infections, nasopharyngitis, arthralgias, and infections [23, 24]. Cases of non-melanoma skin cancers and reversible posterior leukoencephalopathy syndrome (RPLS) have been reported but are quite rare [46]. No internal malignancy risk has been reported or observed with long-term use of ustekinumab. Ustekinumab's overall safety is further supported by a small cohort study demonstrating its safe use during conception and pregnancy with no major patient or fetal adverse events reported [47]. Therefore, ustekinumab is considered a second-line biologic treatment option for use during pregnancy after certolizumab, which is the clear preferred biologic in pregnancy due to its PEGylated structure and lack of the Fc receptor, thereby preventing transfer across the placenta [48].

The most common side effects of guselkumab, tildrakizumab, and risankizumab resemble that of ustekinumab: upper respiratory tract infections, nasopharyngitis, and headaches [31, 32, 39]. Mucocutaneous candidiasis was infrequent and not significantly increased compared to healthy control subjects. Similarly, the rate of new-onset IBD or worsening GI symptoms in patients with psoriasis and IBD were not increased. The lack of mucocutaneous candidiasis or worsening of IBD symptoms with selective IL-23p19 inhibition gives this medication class an edge over the IL-17 antagonists, which have been associated with both adverse events. Long-term studies evaluating the impact of IL-23 blockage and its effect on the GI system are needed and will shed further light on the biological role for IL-23 and IL-17 signaling in the gut.

Future Directions and Summary

The dramatic improvements we have observed in plaque psoriasis with dual inhibition of IL-12/IL-23 and, more recently, selective inhibition of IL-23 via the p19 subunit have been remarkable and provide practitioners with a new class of highly effective medications. Both IL-23 inhibitor classes have shown remarkable safety and durability with continuous treatment. IL-23 antagonists and their respective clinical trials underscore the importance of this cytokine in the pathogenesis of psoriasis and have uncovered some of the differences between IL-23- and IL-17-mediated effects in human health. Nevertheless, some important psoriasis research gaps and unanswered questions remain. For example, we have yet to uncover the exact biological reasons for primary and secondary treatment failures with existing biologic agents in patients with psoriatic disease. We are also unable to accurately predict which specific biologic agent or medication class will be most effective in a patient with psoriasis, thus forcing providers to practice "trial and error" medicine that is largely dictated by insurance coverage and preferred formulary options. We are just now beginning to identify molecular and/or genetic markers that have the potential to guide a more *personalized* approach to psoriasis care. Additionally, the idea that IL-23 is the "master regulator" of psoriatic disease is being challenged by recent, unparalleled efficacy data from phase 2 and 3 clinical trials with dual inhibition of IL-17A/F via bimekizumab [49–53]; this shifts the attention back to the central pathogenic effects of IL-17 on keratinocytes and the feed-forward inflammatory loop it sustains [22]. Finally, the clinical successes we have witnessed for the treatment of plaque psoriasis have clearly outpaced the advances we have made in psoriatic arthritis raising the question as to whether or not IL-23/17 signaling is truly the central immune signal driving psoriatic arthritis versus predominant driver of joint disease in psoriasis patients versus the possibility of other IL-23-independent pathways as predominant disease drivers. For this reason, the complete clinical trial data for the effectiveness of IL-23 antagonists in the treatment of psoriatic arthritis beyond guselkumab is highly anticipated and will add to our overall understanding of the immunologic relationship between plaque psoriasis and other psoriatic variants.

References

1. Griffiths CEM, Armstrong AW, Gudjonsson JE, Barker J. Psoriasis. Lancet. 2021;397(10281):1301–15. https://doi.org/10.1016/S0140-6736(20)32549-6.
2. Takeshita J, Grewal S, Langan SM, Mehta NN, Ogdie A, Van Voorhees AS, et al. Psoriasis and comorbid diseases: epidemiology. J Am Acad Dermatol. 2017;76(3):377–90. https://doi.org/10.1016/j.jaad.2016.07.064.
3. Armstrong AW, Mehta MD, Schupp CW, Gondo GC, Bell SJ, Griffiths CEM. Psoriasis prevalence in adults in the United States. JAMA Dermatol. 2021. doi: https://doi.org/10.1001/jamadermatol.2021.2007.
4. Hawkes JE, Yan BY, Chan TC, Krueger JG. Discovery of the IL-23/IL-17 signaling pathway and the treatment of psoriasis. J Immunol. 2018;201(6):1605–13. https://doi.org/10.4049/jimmunol.1800013.

5. Eedy DJ, Burrows D, Bridges JM, Jones FG. Clearance of severe psoriasis after allogenic bone marrow transplantation. BMJ. 1990;300(6729):908. https://doi.org/10.1136/bmj.300.6729.908.
6. Ellis CN, Gorsulowsky DC, Hamilton TA, Billings JK, Brown MD, Headington JT, et al. Cyclosporine improves psoriasis in a double-blind study. JAMA. 1986;256(22):3110–6.
7. Griffiths CE, Powles AV, Leonard JN, Fry L, Baker BS, Valdimarsson H. Clearance of psoriasis with low dose cyclosporin. Br Med J (Clin Res Ed). 1986;293(6549):731–2. https://doi.org/10.1136/bmj.293.6549.731.
8. Ryan TJ, Baker H. Systemic corticosteroids and folic acid antagonists in the treatment of generalized pustular psoriasis. Evaluation and prognosis based on the study of 104 cases. Br J Dermatol. 1969;81(2):134–45. https://doi.org/10.1111/j.1365-2133.1969.tb15995.x.
9. Gottlieb SL, Gilleaudeau P, Johnson R, Estes L, Woodworth TG, Gottlieb AB, et al. Response of psoriasis to a lymphocyte-selective toxin (DAB389IL-2) suggests a primary immune, but not keratinocyte, pathogenic basis. Nat Med. 1995;1(5):442–7. https://doi.org/10.1038/nm0595-442.
10. Abrams JR, Lebwohl MG, Guzzo CA, Jegasothy BV, Goldfarb MT, Goffe BS, et al. CTLA4Ig-mediated blockade of T-cell costimulation in patients with psoriasis vulgaris. J Clin Invest. 1999;103(9):1243–52. https://doi.org/10.1172/JCI5857.
11. Krueger GG, Callis KP. Development and use of alefacept to treat psoriasis. J Am Acad Dermatol. 2003;49(2 Suppl):S87–97. https://doi.org/10.1016/mjd.2003.552.
12. Lebwohl M, Tyring SK, Hamilton TK, Toth D, Glazer S, Tawfik NH, et al. A novel targeted T-cell modulator, efalizumab, for plaque psoriasis. N Engl J Med. 2003;349(21):2004–13. https://doi.org/10.1056/NEJMoa030002.
13. Oh CJ, Das KM, Gottlieb AB. Treatment with anti-tumor necrosis factor alpha (TNF-alpha) monoclonal antibody dramatically decreases the clinical activity of psoriasis lesions. J Am Acad Dermatol. 2000;42(5 Pt 1):829–30. https://doi.org/10.1067/mjd.2000.105948.
14. Oppmann B, Lesley R, Blom B, Timans JC, Xu Y, Hunte B, et al. Novel p19 protein engages IL-12p40 to form a cytokine, IL-23, with biological activities similar as well as distinct from IL-12. Immunity. 2000;13(5):715–25. https://doi.org/10.1016/s1074-7613(00)00070-4.
15. Kagami S, Rizzo HL, Kurtz SE, Miller LS, Blauvelt A. IL-23 and IL-17A, but not IL-12 and IL-22, are required for optimal skin host defense against Candida albicans. J Immunol. 2010;185(9):5453–62. https://doi.org/10.4049/jimmunol.1001153.
16. Aggarwal S, Ghilardi N, Xie MH, de Sauvage FJ, Gurney AL. Interleukin-23 promotes a distinct CD4 T cell activation state characterized by the production of interleukin-17. J Biol Chem. 2003;278(3):1910–4. https://doi.org/10.1074/jbc.M207577200.
17. Constantinescu CS, Wysocka M, Hilliard B, Ventura ES, Lavi E, Trinchieri G, et al. Antibodies against IL-12 prevent superantigen-induced and spontaneous relapses of experimental autoimmune encephalomyelitis. J Immunol. 1998;161(9):5097–104.
18. Cua DJ, Sherlock J, Chen Y, Murphy CA, Joyce B, Seymour B, et al. Interleukin-23 rather than interleukin-12 is the critical cytokine for autoimmune inflammation of the brain. Nature. 2003;421(6924):744–8. https://doi.org/10.1038/nature01355.
19. Lowes MA, Kikuchi T, Fuentes-Duculan J, Cardinale I, Zaba LC, Haider AS, et al. Psoriasis vulgaris lesions contain discrete populations of Th1 and Th17 T cells. J Invest Dermatol. 2008;128(5):1207–11. https://doi.org/10.1038/sj.jid.5701213.
20. Haider AS, Lowes MA, Suarez-Farinas M, Zaba LC, Cardinale I, Khatcherian A, et al. Identification of cellular pathways of "type 1," Th17 T cells, and TNF- and inducible nitric oxide synthase-producing dendritic cells in autoimmune inflammation through pharmacogenomic study of cyclosporine A in psoriasis. J Immunol. 2008;180(3):1913–20.
21. Lee E, Trepicchio WL, Oestreicher JL, Pittman D, Wang F, Chamian F, et al. Increased expression of interleukin 23 p19 and p40 in lesional skin of patients with psoriasis vulgaris. J Exp Med. 2004;199(1):125–30. https://doi.org/10.1084/jem.20030451.
22. Hawkes JE, Chan TC, Krueger JG. Psoriasis pathogenesis and the development of novel targeted immune therapies. J Allergy Clin Immunol. 2017;140(3):645–53. https://doi.org/10.1016/j.jaci.2017.07.004.
23. Leonardi CL, Kimball AB, Papp KA, Yeilding N, Guzzo C, Wang Y, et al. Efficacy and safety of ustekinumab, a human interleukin-12/23 monoclonal antibody, in patients with psoriasis: 76-week results from a randomised, double-blind, placebo-controlled trial (PHOENIX 1). Lancet. 2008;371(9625):1665–74. https://doi.org/10.1016/S0140-6736(08)60725-4.
24. Papp KA, Langley RG, Lebwohl M, Krueger GG, Szapary P, Yeilding N, et al. Efficacy and safety of ustekinumab, a human interleukin-12/23 monoclonal antibody, in patients with psoriasis: 52-week results from a randomised, double-blind, placebo-controlled trial (PHOENIX 2). Lancet. 2008;371(9625):1675–84. https://doi.org/10.1016/S0140-6736(08)60726-6.
25. Griffiths CE, Strober BE, van de Kerkhof P, Ho V, Fidelus-Gort R, Yeilding N, et al. Comparison of ustekinumab and etanercept for moderate-to-severe psoriasis. N Engl J Med. 2010;362(2):118–28. https://doi.org/10.1056/NEJMoa0810652.
26. Kimball AB, Gordon KB, Fakharzadeh S, Yeilding N, Szapary PO, Schenkel B, et al. Long-term efficacy of ustekinumab in patients with moderate-to-severe psoriasis: results from the PHOENIX 1 trial through up to 3 years. Br J Dermatol. 2012;166(4):861–72. https://doi.org/10.1111/j.1365-2133.2012.10901.x.
27. Landells I, Marano C, Hsu MC, Li S, Zhu Y, Eichenfield LF, et al. Ustekinumab in adolescent patients age 12 to 17 years with moderate-to-severe plaque psoriasis:

results of the randomized phase 3 CADMUS study. J Am Acad Dermatol. 2015;73(4):594–603. https://doi.org/10.1016/j.jaad.2015.07.002.
28. McInnes IB, Kavanaugh A, Gottlieb AB, Puig L, Rahman P, Ritchlin C, et al. Efficacy and safety of ustekinumab in patients with active psoriatic arthritis: 1 year results of the phase 3, multicentre, double-blind, placebo-controlled PSUMMIT 1 trial. Lancet. 2013;382(9894):780–9. https://doi.org/10.1016/S0140-6736(13)60594-2.
29. Ritchlin C, Rahman P, Kavanaugh A, McInnes IB, Puig L, Li S, et al. Efficacy and safety of the anti-IL-12/23 p40 monoclonal antibody, ustekinumab, in patients with active psoriatic arthritis despite conventional non-biological and biological anti-tumour necrosis factor therapy: 6-month and 1-year results of the phase 3, multicentre, double-blind, placebo-controlled, randomised PSUMMIT 2 trial. Ann Rheum Dis. 2014;73(6):990–9. https://doi.org/10.1136/annrheumdis-2013-204655.
30. Kulig P, Musiol S, Freiberger SN, Schreiner B, Gyulveszi G, Russo G, et al. IL-12 protects from psoriasiform skin inflammation. Nat Commun. 2016;7:13466. https://doi.org/10.1038/ncomms13466.
31. Blauvelt A, Papp KA, Griffiths CE, Randazzo B, Wasfi Y, Shen YK, et al. Efficacy and safety of guselkumab, an anti-interleukin-23 monoclonal antibody, compared with adalimumab for the continuous treatment of patients with moderate to severe psoriasis: results from the phase III, double-blinded, placebo- and active comparator-controlled VOYAGE 1 trial. J Am Acad Dermatol. 2017;76(3):405–17. https://doi.org/10.1016/j.jaad.2016.11.041.
32. Reich K, Armstrong AW, Foley P, Song M, Wasfi Y, Randazzo B, et al. Efficacy and safety of guselkumab, an anti-interleukin-23 monoclonal antibody, compared with adalimumab for the treatment of patients with moderate to severe psoriasis with randomized withdrawal and retreatment: results from the phase III, double-blind, placebo- and active comparator-controlled VOYAGE 2 trial. J Am Acad Dermatol. 2017;76(3):418–31. https://doi.org/10.1016/j.jaad.2016.11.042.
33. Langley RG, Tsai TF, Flavin S, Song M, Randazzo B, Wasfi Y, et al. Efficacy and safety of guselkumab in patients with psoriasis who have an inadequate response to ustekinumab: results of the randomized, double-blind, phase III NAVIGATE trial. Br J Dermatol. 2018;178(1):114–23. https://doi.org/10.1111/bjd.15750.
34. Reich K, Armstrong AW, Langley RG, Flavin S, Randazzo B, Li S, et al. Guselkumab versus secukinumab for the treatment of moderate-to-severe psoriasis (ECLIPSE): results from a phase 3, randomised controlled trial. Lancet. 2019;394(10201):831–9. https://doi.org/10.1016/S0140-6736(19)31773-8.
35. Blauvelt A, Papp K, Gottlieb A, Jarell A, Reich K, Maari C, et al. A head-to-head comparison of ixekizumab vs. guselkumab in patients with moderate-to-severe plaque psoriasis: 12-week efficacy, safety and speed of response from a randomized, double-blinded trial. Br J Dermatol. 2020;182(6):1348–58. https://doi.org/10.1111/bjd.18851.
36. Blauvelt A, Leonardi C, Elewski B, Crowley JJ, Guenther LC, Gooderham M, et al. A head-to-head comparison of ixekizumab vs. guselkumab in patients with moderate-to-severe plaque psoriasis: 24-week efficacy and safety results from a randomized, double-blinded trial. Br J Dermatol. 2021;184(6):1047–58. https://doi.org/10.1111/bjd.19509.
37. Deodhar A, Helliwell PS, Boehncke WH, Kollmeier AP, Hsia EC, Subramanian RA, et al. Guselkumab in patients with active psoriatic arthritis who were biologic-naive or had previously received TNFalpha inhibitor treatment (DISCOVER-1): a double-blind, randomised, placebo-controlled phase 3 trial. Lancet. 2020;395(10230):1115–25. https://doi.org/10.1016/S0140-6736(20)30265-8.
38. Mease PJ, Rahman P, Gottlieb AB, Kollmeier AP, Hsia EC, Xu XL, et al. Guselkumab in biologic-naive patients with active psoriatic arthritis (DISCOVER-2): a double-blind, randomised, placebo-controlled phase 3 trial. Lancet. 2020;395(10230):1126–36. https://doi.org/10.1016/S0140-6736(20)30263-4.
39. Reich K, Papp KA, Blauvelt A, Tyring SK, Sinclair R, Thaci D, et al. Tildrakizumab versus placebo or etanercept for chronic plaque psoriasis (reSURFACE 1 and reSURFACE 2): results from two randomised controlled, phase 3 trials. Lancet. 2017;390(10091):276–88. https://doi.org/10.1016/S0140-6736(17)31279-5.
40. Thaci D, Piaserico S, Warren RB, Gupta AK, Cantrell W, Draelos Z, et al. Five-year efficacy and safety of tildrakizumab in patients with moderate-to-severe psoriasis who respond at week 28: pooled analyses of two randomized phase III clinical trials (reSURFACE 1 and reSURFACE 2). Br J Dermatol. 2021;185(2):323–34. https://doi.org/10.1111/bjd.19866.
41. Wu JJ, Jia X, Zhao Y, Carrico J, Brodtkorb TH, Mendelsohn A, et al. Comparative cost-effectiveness of tildrakizumab and other commonly used treatments for moderate-to-severe psoriasis. J Dermatolog Treat. 2020:1–8. https://doi.org/10.1080/09546634.2019.1698700.
42. Gordon KB, Strober B, Lebwohl M, Augustin M, Blauvelt A, Poulin Y, et al. Efficacy and safety of risankizumab in moderate-to-severe plaque psoriasis (UltIMMa-1 and UltIMMa-2): results from two double-blind, randomised, placebo-controlled and ustekinumab-controlled phase 3 trials. Lancet. 2018;392(10148):650–61. https://doi.org/10.1016/S0140-6736(18)31713-6.
43. Reich K, Gooderham M, Thaci D, Crowley JJ, Ryan C, Krueger JG, et al. Risankizumab compared with adalimumab in patients with moderate-to-severe plaque psoriasis (IMMvent): a randomised, double-blind, active-comparator-controlled phase 3 trial. Lancet. 2019;394(10198):576–86. https://doi.org/10.1016/S0140-6736(19)30952-3.

44. Papp KA, Blauvelt A, Bukhalo M, Gooderham M, Krueger JG, Lacour JP, et al. Risankizumab versus Ustekinumab for Moderate-to-Severe Plaque Psoriasis. N Engl J Med. 2017;376(16):1551–60. https://doi.org/10.1056/NEJMoa1607017.
45. Warren RB, Blauvelt A, Poulin Y, Beeck S, Kelly M, Wu T, et al. Efficacy and safety of risankizumab vs. secukinumab in patients with moderate-to-severe plaque psoriasis (IMMerge): results from a phase III, randomized, open-label, efficacy-assessor-blinded clinical trial. Br J Dermatol. 2021;184(1):50–9. https://doi.org/10.1111/bjd.19341.
46. Gottlieb A, Narang K. Ustekinumab in the treatment of psoriatic arthritis: latest findings and clinical potential. Ther Adv Musculoskelet Dis. 2013;5(5):277–85. https://doi.org/10.1177/1759720X13501021.
47. Watson N, Wu K, Farr P, Reynolds NJ, Hampton PJ. Ustekinumab exposure during conception and pregnancy in patients with chronic plaque psoriasis: a case series of 10 pregnancies. Br J Dermatol. 2019;180(1):195–6. https://doi.org/10.1111/bjd.17086.
48. Mariette X, Forger F, Abraham B, Flynn AD, Molto A, Flipo RM, et al. Lack of placental transfer of certolizumab pegol during pregnancy: results from CRIB, a prospective, postmarketing, pharmacokinetic study. Ann Rheum Dis. 2018;77(2):228–33. https://doi.org/10.1136/annrheumdis-2017-212196.
49. Adams R, Maroof A, Baker T, Lawson ADG, Oliver R, Paveley R, et al. Bimekizumab, a novel humanized IgG1 antibody that neutralizes both IL-17A and IL-17F. Front Immunol. 2020;11:1894. https://doi.org/10.3389/fimmu.2020.01894.
50. Gordon KB, Foley P, Krueger JG, Pinter A, Reich K, Vender R, et al. Bimekizumab efficacy and safety in moderate to severe plaque psoriasis (BE READY): a multicentre, double-blind, placebo-controlled, randomised withdrawal phase 3 trial. Lancet. 2021;397(10273):475–86. https://doi.org/10.1016/S0140-6736(21)00126-4.
51. Reich K, Papp KA, Blauvelt A, Langley RG, Armstrong A, Warren RB, et al. Bimekizumab versus ustekinumab for the treatment of moderate to severe plaque psoriasis (BE VIVID): efficacy and safety from a 52-week, multicentre, double-blind, active comparator and placebo controlled phase 3 trial. Lancet. 2021;397(10273):487–98. https://doi.org/10.1016/S0140-6736(21)00125-2.
52. Reich K, Warren RB, Lebwohl M, Gooderham M, Strober B, Langley RG, et al. Bimekizumab versus Secukinumab in Plaque Psoriasis. N Engl J Med. 2021;385(2):142–52. https://doi.org/10.1056/NEJMoa2102383.
53. Warren RB, Blauvelt A, Bagel J, Papp KA, Yamauchi P, Armstrong A, et al. Bimekizumab versus Adalimumab in Plaque Psoriasis. N Engl J Med. 2021;385(2):130–41. https://doi.org/10.1056/NEJMoa2102388.

Combination Therapy with Biologic Agents

6

Kourtney Pony and Mio Nakamura

Introduction

Long-term remission of psoriasis can be difficult to achieve due to the waxing and waning nature of this chronic systemic inflammatory condition. With the advent of various biologic agents for the treatment of moderate-to-severe psoriasis, it is now possible for many patients to achieve adequate disease control with subsequent improvement in quality of life [1]. However, in some circumstances, combining a biologic agent with one or more additional therapeutic agents may be necessary to maintain adequate disease control. Such patients may include those with only partial response to monotherapy, those whose psoriasis worsens due to loss of efficacy of a treatment over time, or those with comorbidities such as psoriatic arthritis which may not be adequately treated with monotherapy. This chapter will review the existing evidence of various combination therapies with biologic agents for the treatment of psoriasis, specifically the combination of biologic agents with phototherapy, oral systemic agents, and other biologic agents.

K. Pony
University of Michigan Medical School, Ann Arbor, MI, USA

M. Nakamura (✉)
Department of Dermatology, University of Michigan, Ann Arbor, MI, USA
e-mail: mionak@med.umich.edu

Rationale for Combination Therapy

Because psoriasis is a chronic disease with episodic flares, an effective treatment with rapid onset is required for acute flares, while maintenance agents are needed for adequate long-term disease control [2]. In combination therapy, one agent can be used to treat psoriasis acutely, while the safer of the two agents can be used as maintenance treatment [3]. For patients with severe recalcitrant disease, the concomitant use of two or more agents with varying mechanisms of action may increase the overall efficacy of psoriasis therapy in an additive or synergistic manner. Combination therapy may also allow for use of lower doses of each agent to minimize toxicity [4].

Types of Combination Therapy

With the current armamentarium of available psoriasis therapies, there are many opportunities to combine various agents. However, when combining treatments, the provider must be aware of each treatment agent's mechanism of action, safety profile, and drug-drug interactions so that an effective, yet safe, combination therapy can be instituted. For example, caution should be taken to avoid overlapping side effect profiles, such as immunosuppression that can increase risk of malignancy or infection.

N. Brownstone et al. (eds.), *Biologic Therapy for Psoriasis*, Updates in Clinical Dermatology,
https://doi.org/10.1007/978-3-030-92938-1_6

To maximize the efficacy and safety of combination therapy, different techniques in combination therapy have been described for the treatment of psoriasis such as concomitant therapy, rotational therapy, and sequential therapy. In *concomitant therapy*, two or more agents are used simultaneously for synergistic or additive effects. *Rotational therapy* was first described by Weinstein and White in 1993 and rotates available psoriasis treatments every 2–3 years, which minimizes cumulative toxicity by long periods off each treatment [5]. *Sequential therapy*, first described by Koo, uses two or more therapies in a deliberate sequence to optimize therapeutic outcomes, as some psoriasis therapies are better suited for rapid clearance, while others are more appropriate for long-term maintenance [6]. Specifically, sequential therapy consists of three distinct phases as follows: Phase 1, the clearing phase involving the use of a very efficacious, rapidly acting agent, which may have more long-term risks; Phase 2, the transitional phase involving introduction of the maintenance agent and tapering of the rapidly acting agent; and Phase 3, the maintenance phase involving the maintenance agent with less efficacy but better long-term safety profile.

Other Considerations When Prescribing Combination Therapy

In addition to maximizing safety and efficacy, combination therapy must consider patient acceptability and compliance. For example, office-based phototherapy may not be a practical addition to biologic therapy for a patient with limited access to transportation. A needle-phobic patient would not be good candidate for multiple biologic therapies. Furthermore, cost of combination therapy must also be considered. For example, insurance companies will likely be hesitant to approve coverage for two different biologic agents or a biologic agent and apremilast for the same patient. In such instances, the provider may need to go the extra mile and provide adequate medical justification to secure insurance approval or financial assistance so that the patient can receive adequate treatment.

Combining Biologics with Phototherapy

Phototherapy, especially narrowband ultraviolet B (NB-UVB) and excimer laser, can be used safely and effectively with a biologic agent. This combination therapy can be used for patients with recalcitrant psoriasis despite monotherapy with a biologic agent or phototherapy.

Efficacy

Several studies have evaluated the combination regimen of etanercept and NB-UVB and showed that combination therapy was superior to either monotherapy with reduced time to clearance [7–13]. In a 12-week, single-arm, open-label study, the combination of etanercept 50 mg twice weekly and NB-UVB three times weekly was evaluated in 86 patients. PASI-75 (75% improvement or greater in the Psoriasis Area and Severity Index) was achieved in 84.9% of patients at 12 weeks [8]. In another study, eight patients who failed monotherapy with NB-UVB phototherapy followed by monotherapy with etanercept 50 mg twice weekly for 12 weeks were treated with the combination of etanercept and phototherapy [11]. All eight of these patients achieved PASI-75 with the combination regimen. High adherence to the NB-UVB regimen appears to be important to achieve significant clinical improvement [12]. The addition of excimer laser to etanercept therapy has also been reported to produce effective results when etanercept plus traditional NB-UVB therapy has failed [14]. However, one head-to-head pilot study examining the combination treatment of NB-UVB plus etanercept 50 mg twice weekly failed to show efficacy of combination therapy over monotherapy [15]. This study was limited by a small sample size of 13 patients who all had a body mass index (BMI) of greater than 30, and psoriasis patients with a BMI of greater than 30 have been shown to have suboptimal response to etanercept [16].

There have been several studies investigating the combination of adalimumab and phototherapy [13, 17–19]. In a 24-week, single-arm, open-label study by Bagel, 85% (17/20) of patients were clear or almost clear at 12 weeks of combination treatment with adalimumab and NB-UVB [17]. In a half-body comparison study of patients on adalimumab, Wolf et al. found overall mean PASI reduction from baseline of 86% on UV-irradiated body halves vs. 53% on nonirradiated body halves [18]. These studies demonstrated that phototherapy significantly accelerates therapeutic response and improves the clearance of psoriatic lesions in patients treated with adalimumab [17–19].

One study to date has evaluated the combination of ustekinumab plus NB-UVB [20]. This intraindividual, half-body comparison study showed that PASI-75 was achieved significantly more often on the UV-irradiated half than on the nonirradiated half at week 6 [20]. A retrospective review of three patients [13] and a case series of two patients [21] also describe the role of adding NB-UVB phototherapy to ustekinumab to achieve better disease control.

Safety

Based on the above studies, the combination of biologics with NB-UVB or excimer laser has acceptable tolerability with limited safety concerns. Rate of adverse events for the combination regimen did not appear to differ from either therapy alone [22]. However, one theoretical safety concern with combining biologic therapy and phototherapy is the increased risk of keratinocyte carcinomas. Biologic monotherapy has been possibly associated with a slightly increased risk of keratinocyte carcinomas [23]. While NB-UVB phototherapy has not been shown to increase the risk of keratinocyte carcinomas, psoralen + ultraviolet A (PUVA) has been shown to increase the risk of squamous cell carcinoma in Caucasian psoriasis patients who have undergone more than 250 PUVA sessions [24]. No studies to date have investigated the combination therapy of biologics and PUVA. Further research is needed to assess long-term skin cancer risk and other adverse events of this combination therapy. Providers should consider close routine follow-up with total body skin examinations for patients on both a biologic agent and phototherapy.

Furthermore, adding phototherapy to an existing biologic therapy may be the safest option for patients with severe psoriasis recalcitrant to biologic monotherapy who are pregnant/lactating. While no studies to date have been specifically conducted in this population, biologic monotherapy and phototherapy can be used safely in pregnancy/lactation. Furthermore, patients who have failed biologic therapy with comorbidities such as liver disease or kidney disease who may not be candidates for traditional systemic therapies such as methotrexate, acitretin, and cyclosporine would also benefit from the addition of phototherapy, which has no systemic adverse effects.

Combining Biologic Agents with Methotrexate

The use of biologic agents, especially tumor necrosis factor-alpha (TNF-alpha) inhibitors, in combination with methotrexate is often used in clinical practice. This combination is frequently used for patients who failed monotherapy with a biologic agent or methotrexate, as well as patients with both psoriasis and psoriatic arthritis [25]. The addition of methotrexate to biologic therapy may also decrease the risk of developing antidrug antibodies (ADAs) or reverse the presence of ADAs [26–28]. Many studies have investigated the combination of methotrexate and TNF-alpha inhibitors etanercept, adalimumab, and infliximab [29–48]. Studies investigating combination of other biologic agents such as interleukin (IL)-12/23, IL-17, and IL-23 agents are limited to date [49, 50].

Efficacy

In a large randomized, double-blind, placebo-controlled study of 239 patients per arm, patients received etanercept alone vs. etanercept plus methotrexate. PASI-75 was significantly higher at weeks 12 and 24 for the combination therapy group compared to the etanercept-only group (70.2% vs. 54.3%, $P = 0.01$, and 77.3% vs. 60.3%, $P < 0.0001$, respectively) [29]. In another study, 31 patients were treated with etanercept plus methotrexate, and 28 patients were treated with initial combination therapy of etanercept plus methotrexate with subsequent taper and discontinuation of methotrexate [30]. After 24 weeks, while both groups showed significant improvement in psoriasis, a significantly greater proportion of patients in the continued combination regimen achieved Physician Global Assessment (PGA) score of "clear" or "almost clear" compared to the taper/discontinuation group [30]. In many patients, improvement achieved during combination therapy with etanercept and methotrexate can be sustained despite gradually tapering off methotrexate [31], or the combination therapy can successfully reduce the required dose of methotrexate [32]. The combination regimen may also allow for faster treatment responses and safe transitioning from one systemic agent to another [33]. The combination of etanercept and methotrexate has also shown to reduce serum levels of IL-17A, IL-23, TNF-α, and their mRNA expression in peripheral blood mononuclear cells (PBMCs) to a greater extent compared to etanercept monotherapy [34]. Similarly, the etanercept biosimilar appears to show better efficacy in combination with methotrexate compared to the biosimilar agent alone [35].

The combination of adalimumab and methotrexate is also commonly used in clinical practice [36] and can be used when insufficient improvement of psoriasis is achieved with adalimumab monotherapy [37]. Furthermore, in a study by De Groot et al., methotrexate or adalimumab monotherapy resulted in downregulation of some inflammatory markers, while skin samples from patients treated with both adalimumab and methotrexate showed downregulation of all inflammatory markers assessed, including CD3, CD68, CD161, elastase, BDCA-2, and TNF-alpha [38], suggesting that combination therapy more effectively reduces inflammation in psoriatic skin.

While studies investigating the long-term effectiveness of the combination therapy of biologic agents with methotrexate are overall limited, two studies have focused on the long-term effects of the combination of infliximab and methotrexate [39, 40]. Dalaker and Bonesrønning retrospectively reviewed the charts of a total of 23 patients treated with infliximab and methotrexate or azathioprine. The longest duration of the combination regimen using infliximab and methotrexate was 5 years and 5 months. They concluded that the combination is safe and effective for long-term use [39]. In another study by Spertino et al., combination of infliximab and methotrexate resulted in increased likelihood of maintaining treatment effectiveness after 1 year of treatment compared to infliximab monotherapy.

With regard to other biologic agents, a retrospective review of 12 patients with moderate-to-severe psoriasis treated with ustekinumab and methotrexate concluded that the combination is effective and well-tolerated [49]. The successful use of IL-17 inhibitors secukinumab and brodalumab in combination with methotrexate has only been reported in case reports in patients with severe psoriasis recalcitrant to multiple monotherapies [50, 51]. Further studies are needed to determine the efficacy, especially long-term efficacy, of combining IL-17 and IL-23 agents with methotrexate.

Safety

Several studies have investigated the safety of combining biologic agents and methotrexate [29, 33, 46], including some long-term studies [39, 40, 52]. Overall, the adverse event profile of the combination therapy appears to be similar to those of the individual agents when used as monotherapy; there appear to be no additional or synergistic adverse events during combination therapy. Regarding long-term safety, in a retrospective study investigating a total of 176 treatments with TNF-alpha inhibitors etanercept or adalimumab with or without methotrexate, Hoffman et al. found that the combination therapy is well-tolerated long-term over an average duration of combination therapy of 76.5 weeks [52]. This study showed that combination therapy with methotrexate resulted in a higher incidence of laboratory abnormalities, but these lab abnormalities were expected possible adverse events of methotrexate monotherapy [52].

Combining Biologic Agents with Acitretin

While large-scale, prospective, controlled studies evaluating the combination of biologic agents plus acitretin are limited, this combination appears to be safe and effective for the treatment of severe psoriasis recalcitrant to either monotherapy. It has been suggested that this combination regimen may be successful for treating recalcitrant psoriasis due to the difference in therapeutic effects of each of these agents; while biologics target the inflammatory pathways implicated in psoriasis, acitretin is thought to be effective for psoriasis due to its antiproliferative effects [53].

Efficacy

In 2 24-week, randomized, controlled, investigator-blinded pilot trials, 60 patients with moderate-to-severe psoriasis were randomized to receive etanercept 25 mg twice weekly, acitretin daily, or etanercept 25 mg once weekly plus acitretin daily. It was found that the combination of etanercept 25 mg once weekly and acitretin is as effective as etanercept 25 mg twice weekly and more effective than acitretin alone [54, 55]. In a retrospective study of five patients treated with anti-TNF-alpha agents etanercept, adalimumab, or infliximab, the combination of the biologic agent and acitretin allowed for significant improvement of severe psoriasis that had previously failed acitretin monotherapy [56]. Adding acitretin also appears to allow for successful dose reduction of etanercept without losing efficacy [57].

The use of ustekinumab in combination with acitretin was summarized in a retrospective review in which five patients were effectively and safely treated with this combination [49]. The data regarding combination therapy of secukinumab and acitretin is limited to a case series of three patients with chronic plaque, generalized pustular, and erythrodermic psoriasis with multiple comorbidities who failed several conventional and biologic therapies including escalated dose regimens of secukinumab. The combination of secukinumab and low-dose acitretin resulted in a complete or almost complete clearance in all patients with no adverse events or increased toxicity [58]. Currently, there are no published reports regarding the combination of other IL-17 agents or IL-23 agents and acitretin.

Safety

In the above studies, the combination of biologics and acitretin was well-tolerated [49, 53–58]. Adverse events and laboratory abnormalities, when they occurred, were consistent with known side effects of monotherapy. Future studies are needed to delineate the long-term safety profile of this combination therapy.

Combining Biologic Agents with Cyclosporine

No large-scale, prospective, controlled studies have been conducted to evaluate the safety and efficacy of combining biologics and cyclosporine, but this combination appears to be beneficial for short-term use in recalcitrant cases of psoriasis [59, 60]. In patients requiring rapid improvement of psoriasis, these two agents may be used in combination initially, with subsequent taper off cyclosporine as the psoriasis improves. Because patients on cyclosporine require an effective long-term treatment regimen, cyclosporine may be overlapped with biologic therapy for several weeks while tapering off cyclosporine [61–65]. The short-term combination of etanercept and cyclosporine may also be used successfully in the pediatric population [66, 67].

Efficacy

In a small prospective study, seven patients with refractory psoriasis were treated with cyclosporine 200 mg per day plus etanercept 50 mg weekly until their psoriasis was clear or near clear [59]. In another study, 11 patients with psoriasis and psoriatic arthritis whose cutaneous manifestations were uncontrolled on etanercept alone received cyclosporine with improvement of their psoriasis [60].

Studies investigating the combination of adalimumab with cyclosporine are limited to patients with psoriatic arthritis [61]. In a prospective 12-month, nonrandomized, unblinded clinical trial of 57, 58, and 55 patients with severely active PsA and inadequate response to MTX who received cyclosporine (2.5–3.75 mg/kg/day), adalimumab (40 mg every other week), or combination, respectively, the combination therapy produced major improvement in both clinical and serological variables [61].

Several studies have described the use of biologic agents and cyclosporine in combination to transition from cyclosporine therapy to biologic therapy. A case series of eight patients describe the successful transition from cyclosporine to long-term treatment with etanercept after 2–4 weeks of combination therapy [62]. A retrospective chart review of ten patients with severe psoriasis on cyclosporine showed successful transition to adalimumab after an average of 10 weeks of combination therapy [63]. Two case reports to date have described the successful transition from cyclosporine to etanercept in the pediatric population [66, 67].

Safety

Long-term consequences of this combination are not well known. In the above studies, the short-term use of the combination of a biologic agent plus cyclosporine was well-tolerated. Adverse events were similar to those seen with monotherapy. Long-term (>2 years) use of cyclosporine has been shown to increase the risk of skin cancer in psoriasis patients [68], and biologic agents, specifically anti-TNF-alpha agents, may also increase the risk of skin cancer [23]. Therefore, the concomitant use of anti-TNF-alpha agents and cyclosporine should be limited to short-term use. The long-term safety of this combination, as well as with other classes of biologic agents, requires further investigation.

Combining Biologics with Apremilast

Only a limited number of retrospective studies and case reports have investigated the combination of biologic agents with apremilast [69–72]. Given that apremilast and biologics have different mechanisms of action and side effect profiles, this combination may be safe and effective in patients with severe recalcitrant psoriasis.

Efficacy

In a retrospective review by AbuHilal et al., 13 patients were treated with a combination of apremilast and an anti-TNF-alpha agent (7 infliximab, 4 etanercept, 2 adalimumab), 7 were treated with apremilast and both methotrexate and a TNF-alpha inhibitor (5 adalimumab and methotrexate, 2 infliximab and methotrexate), and 13 patients were treated with apremilast and ustekinumab. They found that combination therapy of biologics and apremilast may be beneficial in patients who were unable to achieve sufficient disease control with monotherapy or those with decrease in efficacy of monotherapy overtime [69]. Other reports on the use of biologics in combination with apremilast are limited to case reports of adalimumab [70] and secukinumab [71, 72].

Safety

In the above reports, the combination of biologics and apremilast was well-tolerated, with adverse events being those known of apremilast such as gastrointestinal upset, headache, and weight loss [69]. Large-scale, prospective, randomized, long-term studies are needed.

Combining Biologic Agents

The use of more than one biologic agent in combination is reported in several case reports and case series [49, 73–78]. The use of two biologic agents in different classes with different mechanisms of action and side effect profiles may be safe and effective in a select subset of patients with recalcitrant psoriasis with or without psoriatic arthritis and those with comorbidities that prohibit the use of oral systemic medications or phototherapy.

Efficacy

To date, six patients have been treated with ustekinumab and etanercept [49, 73–75, 78], four with ustekinumab and adalimumab [49, 75, 76], and one each with ustekinumab and certolizumab [75], ustekinumab and golimumab [75], secukinumab and etanercept [78], guselkumab and etanercept [78], and guselkumab and adalimumab [77], with effective disease control.

Safety

The use of biologic agents in combination may lead to greater immunosuppression, theoretically increasing the risk of infection or malignancy. The potential risks and benefits of combination therapy should be considered and discussed with the patient prior to initiation of this treatment regimen. Further studies are needed to delineate the safety and efficacy of combining multiple biologic agents.

Conclusion

The currently available data supports the use of combination therapy in various circumstances to manage difficult-to-treat psoriasis. While further investigations are needed to gain further knowledge of the long-term safety and efficacy of various combination therapies, providers should consider combining various treatment modalities to maximize efficacy of treatments while maintaining a favorable safety profile. An individualized approach should be taken that considers the individual patient's treatment goals, comorbidities, and social circumstances.

References

1. Bhutani T, Patel T, Koo B, Nguyen T, Hong J, Koo J. A prospective, interventional assessment of psoriasis quality of life using a nonskin-specific validated instrument that allows comparison with other major medical conditions. J Am Acad Dermatol. 2013;69(2):e79–88. https://doi.org/10.1016/j.jaad.2012.10.009.
2. Emer J, Lebwohl MG. Combination, rotational, and sequential therapies. In: Koo JYM, Levin EC, Leon A, Wu JJ, Gottlieb AB, editors. Moderate to severe psoriasis. Boca Raton: CRC Press; 2015. p. 121–38.
3. Lebwohl M, Menter A, Koo J, Feldman SR. Combination therapy to treat moderate to severe psoriasis. J Am Acad Dermatol. 2004;50(3):416–30. https://doi.org/10.1016/j.jaad.2002.12.002.
4. Menter MA, See JA, Amend WJ, Ellis CN, Krueger GG, Lebwohl M, et al. Proceedings of the psoriasis combination and rotation therapy conference. Deer Valley, Utah, Oct. 7–9, 1994. J Am Acad Dermatol. 1996;34(2 Pt 1):315–21. https://doi.org/10.1016/s0190-9622(96)80148-4. Erratum in: J Am Acad Dermatol 1996 Jun;34(6):1029.
5. Weinstein GD, White GM. An approach to the treatment of moderate to severe psoriasis with rotational therapy. J Am Acad Dermatol. 1993;28(3):454–9. https://doi.org/10.1016/0190-9622(93)70067-4.
6. Koo J. Systemic sequential therapy of psoriasis: a new paradigm for improved therapeutic results. J Am Acad Dermatol. 1999;41(3 Pt 2):S25–8. https://doi.org/10.1016/s0190-9622(99)70363-4.

7. De Simone C, D'Agostino M, Capizzi R, Capponi A, Venier A, Caldarola G. Combined treatment with etanercept 50 mg once weekly and narrow-band ultraviolet B phototherapy in chronic plaque psoriasis. Eur J Dermatol. 2011;21(4):568–72. https://doi.org/10.1684/ejd.2011.1330.
8. Kircik L, Bagel J, Korman N, Menter A, Elmets CA, Koo J, et al. Utilization of narrow-band ultraviolet light B therapy and etanercept for the treatment of psoriasis (UNITE): efficacy, safety, and patient-reported outcomes. J Drugs Dermatol. 2008;7(3):245–53.
9. Wolf P, Hofer A, Legat FJ, et al. Treatment with 311-nm ultraviolet B accelerates and improves the clearance of psoriatic lesions in patients treated with etanercept. Br J Dermatol. 2009;160(1):186–9. https://doi.org/10.1111/j.1365-2133.2008.08926.x.
10. Gambichler T, Tigges C, Scola N, et al. Etanercept plus narrowband ultraviolet B phototherapy of psoriasis is more effective than etanercept monotherapy at 6 weeks. Br J Dermatol. 2011;164(6):1383–6. https://doi.org/10.1111/j.1365-2133.2011.10358.x.
11. Calzavara-Pinton PG, Sala R, Arisi M, Rossi MT, Venturini M, Ortel B. Synergism between narrowband ultraviolet B phototherapy and etanercept for the treatment of plaque-type psoriasis. Br J Dermatol. 2013;169(1):130–6. https://doi.org/10.1111/bjd.12277. PMID: 23834117.
12. Lynde CW, Gupta AK, Guenther L, et al. A randomized study comparing the combination of nbUVB and etanercept to etanercept monotherapy in patients with psoriasis who do not exhibit an excellent response after 12 weeks of etanercept. J Dermatolog Treat. 2012;23(4):261–7. https://doi.org/10.3109/09546634.2011.607795.
13. Belinchón I, Arribas MP, Soro P, Betlloch I. Recovery of the response to biological treatments using narrow band ultraviolet-B in patients with moderate to severe psoriasis: a retrospective study of 17 patients. Photodermatol Photoimmunol Photomed. 2014;30(6):316–22. https://doi.org/10.1111/phpp.12134. PMID: 25132192.
14. Park KK, Swan J, Koo J. Effective treatment of etanercept and phototherapy-resistant psoriasis using the excimer laser. Dermatol Online J. 2012;18(3):2.
15. Park KK, Wu JJ, Koo J. A randomized, 'head-to-head' pilot study comparing the effects of etanercept monotherapy vs. etanercept and narrowband ultraviolet B (NB-UVB) phototherapy in obese psoriasis patients. J Eur Acad Dermatol Venereol. 2013;27(7):899–906. https://doi.org/10.1111/j.1468-3083.2012.04611.x.
16. Strober B, Gottlieb A, Leonardi C, et al. Levels of response of psoriasis patients with different baseline characteristics treated with etanercept. J Am Acad Dermatol. 2006;54(3 Suppl):AB220.
17. Bagel J. Adalimumab plus narrowband ultraviolet B light phototherapy for the treatment of moderate to severe psoriasis. J Drugs Dermatol. 2011;10(4):366–71.
18. Wolf P, Hofer A, Weger W, Posch-Fabian T, Gruber-Wackernagel A, Legat FJ. 311 nm ultraviolet B-accelerated response of psoriatic lesions in adalimumab-treated patients. Photodermatol Photoimmunol Photomed. 2011;27(4):86–9. https://doi.org/10.1111/j.1600-0781.2011.00594.x.
19. Lucas A, Belinchón I, Pérez-Crespo M, Mataix J, Betlloch I. Successful response to narrow-band UVB in a patient undergoing concomitant treatment with adalimumab for psoriasis. Australas J Dermatol. 2008;49(3):173–4. https://doi.org/10.1111/j.1440-0960.2008.00458.x.
20. Wolf P, Weger W, Legat FJ, et al. Treatment with 311-nm ultraviolet B enhanced response of psoriatic lesions in ustekinumab-treated patients: a randomized intraindividual trial. Br J Dermatol. 2012;166(1):147–53. https://doi.org/10.1111/j.1365-2133.2011.10616.x.
21. Soro Martínez P, Belinchón Romero I, Arribas Granados MP. Restoration of response to ustekinumab with narrowband UV-B phototherapy. Actas Dermosifiliogr. 2014;105(2):200–2. https://doi.org/10.1016/j.ad.2013.03.007.
22. Farahnik B, Patel V, Beroukhim K, Zhu TH, Abrouk M, Nakamura M, et al. Combining biologic and phototherapy treatments for psoriasis: safety, efficacy, and patient acceptability. Psoriasis (Auckl). 2016;6:105–11. https://doi.org/10.2147/PTT.S98952.
23. Patel RV, Clark LN, Lebwohl M, Weinberg JM. Treatments for psoriasis and the risk of malignancy. J Am Acad Dermatol. 2009;60(6):1001–17. https://doi.org/10.1016/j.jaad.2008.12.031.
24. Wang E, Sasaki J, Nakamura M, Koo J. Cutaneous carcinogenic risk of phototherapy: an updated comprehensive review. J Psoriasis Psoriatic Arthritis. 2016;1:44–51.
25. Bonomo L, Abittan BJ, Hashim PW, Karki C, Mason M, Lebwohl M. Combination use of systemic therapies in psoriasis: baseline characteristics from the Corrona Psoriasis Registry. J Drugs Dermatol. 2019;18(8):731–40.
26. Adişen E, Aral A, Aybay C, Gürer MA. Anti-infliximab antibody status and its relation to clinical response in psoriatic patients: a pilot study. J Dermatol. 2010;37(8):708–13. https://doi.org/10.1111/j.1346-8138.2010.00882.x.
27. Vincent T, Best M, Plawecki M, Girard C. Complete reversion of anti-infliximab immunization by methotrexate combination in a patient with psoriasis. J Dermatol. 2015;42(10):1030–1. https://doi.org/10.1111/1346-8138.13010.
28. Farhangian ME, Feldman SR. Immunogenicity of biologic treatments for psoriasis: therapeutic consequences and the potential value of concomitant methotrexate. Am J Clin Dermatol. 2015;16(4):285–94. https://doi.org/10.1007/s40257-015-0131-y.
29. Gottlieb AB, Langley RG, Strober BE, Papp KA, Klekotka P, Creamer K, et al. A randomized, double-blind, placebo-controlled study to evaluate the addition of methotrexate to etanercept in patients with moderate to severe plaque psoriasis. Br J Dermatol. 2012;167(3):649–57. https://doi.org/10.1111/j.1365-2133.2012.11015.x.

30. Zachariae C, Mørk NJ, Reunala T, et al. The combination of etanercept and methotrexate increases the effectiveness of treatment in active psoriasis despite inadequate effect of methotrexate therapy. Acta Derm Venereol. 2008;88(5):495–501. https://doi.org/10.2340/00015555-0511.
31. Yamauchi PS, Lowe NJ. Etanercept therapy allows the tapering of methotrexate and sustained clinical responses in patients with moderate to severe psoriasis. Int J Dermatol. 2008;47(2):202–4. https://doi.org/10.1111/j.1365-4632.2008.03419.x.
32. Sherman S, Hodak E, Pavlovsky L. Can etanercept treatment failure in moderate-to-severe psoriasis be overcome by addition of low-dose methotrexate? A single-center experience. J Dermatolog Treat. 2018;29(7):666–70. https://doi.org/10.1080/09546634.2018.1441491.
33. Foley PA, Quirk C, Sullivan JR, Dolianitis C, Hack SP, Thirunavukkarasu K, et al. Combining etanercept with traditional agents in the treatment of psoriasis: a review of the clinical evidence. J Eur Acad Dermatol Venereol. 2010;24(10):1135–43. https://doi.org/10.1111/j.1468-3083.2010.03613.x.
34. Yu Q, Tong Y, Cui L, Zhang L, Gong Y, Diao H, Gao F, Shi Y. Efficacy and safety of etanercept combined plus methotrexate and comparison of expression of pro-inflammatory factors expression for the treatment of moderate-to-severe plaque psoriasis. Int Immunopharmacol. 2019;73:442–50. https://doi.org/10.1016/j.intimp.2019.05.042.
35. Liu LF, Chen JS, Gu J, Xu JH, Jin HZ, Pang XW, et al. Etanercept biosimilar (recombinant human tumor necrosis factor-α receptor II: IgG Fc fusion protein) and methotrexate combination therapy in Chinese patients with moderate-to-severe plaque psoriasis: a multicentre, randomized, double-blind, placebo-controlled trial. Arch Dermatol Res. 2020;312(6):437–45. https://doi.org/10.1007/s00403-019-02024-6.
36. Philipp S, Wilsmann-Theis D, Weyergraf A, Rotterdam S, Frambach Y, Gerdes S, et al. Combination of adalimumab with traditional systemic antipsoriatic drugs - a report of 39 cases. J Dtsch Dermatol Ges. 2012;10(11):821–37. https://doi.org/10.1111/j.1610-0387.2012.07976.x.
37. van den Reek JM, van Lümig PP, Kievit W, Zweegers J, van de Kerkhof PC, Seyger MM, et al. Effectiveness of adalimumab dose escalation, combination therapy of adalimumab with methotrexate, or both in patients with psoriasis in daily practice. J Dermatolog Treat. 2013;24(5):361–8. https://doi.org/10.3109/09546634.2012.751483.
38. De Groot M, Teunissen MBM, Picavet DI, Wolbink GJ, Tal P, de Rie M, et al. Adalimumab in combination with methotrexate more effectively reduces the numbers of different inflammatory cell types in lesional psoriatic skin than does single treatment with adalimumab or methotrexate. Br J Dermatol. 2008;159:1401.
39. Dalaker M, Bonesrønning JH. Long-term maintenance treatment of moderate-to-severe plaque psoriasis with infliximab in combination with methotrexate or azathioprine in a retrospective cohort. J Eur Acad Dermatol Venereol. 2009;23(3):277–82. https://doi.org/10.1111/j.1468-3083.2008.03039.
40. Spertino J, Lopez-Ferrer A, Vilarrasa E, Puig L. Long-term study of infliximab for psoriasis in daily practice: drug survival depends on combined treatment, obesity and infusion reactions. J Eur Acad Dermatol Venereol. 2014;28(11):1514–21. https://doi.org/10.1111/jdv.12331.
41. Driessen RJ, van de Kerkhof PC, de Jong EM. Etanercept combined with methotrexate for high-need psoriasis. Br J Dermatol. 2008;159(2):460–3. https://doi.org/10.1111/j.1365-2133.2008.08669.x.
42. Iyer S, Yamauchi P, Lowe NJ. Etanercept for severe psoriasis and psoriatic arthritis: observations on combination therapy. Br J Dermatol. 2002;146(1):118–21.
43. Strober BE, Clarke S. Etanercept for the treatment of psoriasis: combination therapy with other modalities. J Drugs Dermatol. 2004;3(3):270–2. https://doi.org/10.1046/j.0007-0963.2001.04529.x.
44. Muñoz-Santos C, Vidal D, Gomez-Vazquez M, Sola-Ortigosa J, Guilabert A. Etanercept and methotrexate combination therapy for the treatment of moderate to severe psoriasis: a retrospective multicentre study. Australas J Dermatol. 2016;57(4):e147–8. https://doi.org/10.1111/ajd.12495.
45. Atzeni F, Boccassini L, Antivalle M, Salaffi F, Sarzi-Puttini P. Etanercept plus ciclosporin versus etanercept plus methotrexate for maintaining clinical control over psoriatic arthritis: a randomised pilot study. Ann Rheum Dis. 2011;70(4):712–4. https://doi.org/10.1136/ard.2010.130864.
46. Babino G, Giunta A, Ruzzetti M, Sole Chimenti M, Chimenti S, Esposito M. Combination therapy with etanercept in psoriasis: retrospective analysis of efficacy and safety outcomes from real-life practice. J Int Med Res. 2016;44(1 suppl):100–5. https://doi.org/10.1177/0300060515593260.
47. Takeshita J, Wang S, Shin DB, Callis Duffin K, Krueger GG, Kalb RE, et al. Comparative effectiveness of less commonly used systemic monotherapies and common combination therapies for moderate to severe psoriasis in the clinical setting. J Am Acad Dermatol. 2014;71(6):1167–75. https://doi.org/10.1016/j.jaad.2014.08.003.
48. Busard CI, Cohen AD, Wolf P, Gkalpakiotis S, Cazzaniga S, Stern RS, et al. Biologics combined with conventional systemic agents or phototherapy for the treatment of psoriasis: real-life data from PSONET registries. J Eur Acad Dermatol Venereol. 2018;32(2):245–53. https://doi.org/10.1111/jdv.14583.
49. Heinecke GM, Luber AJ, Levitt JO, Lebwohl MG. Combination use of ustekinumab with other systemic therapies: a retrospective study in a tertiary referral center. J Drugs Dermatol. 2013;12(10):1098–102.
50. Kostaki D, Aquila E, Macaluso L, Mattozzi C, Richetta AG. Optimizing secukinumab treatment in psoriasis with concomitant methotrexate admin-

istration: minireview and a case report. Case Rep Dermatol. 2019;11(Suppl 1):17–22. https://doi.org/10.1159/000501994.
51. Armesto S, González Vela C, Sánchez J, Illaro A, Mayorga J, López Sundh AE, et al. Treating multidrug-resistant psoriasis with brodalumab, apremilast, methotrexate and prednisone combination therapy in the COVID-19 pandemic. Dermatol Ther. 2020;33(6):e14464. https://doi.org/10.1111/dth.14464.
52. Hoffmann JHO, Knoop C, Schäkel K, Enk AH, Hadaschik EN. Long-term safety of combination treatment with methotrexate and tumor necrosis factor (TNF)-α antagonists versus TNF-α antagonists alone in psoriatic patients. J Dermatol. 2021;48(6):835–43. https://doi.org/10.1111/1346-8138.15754.
53. Conley J, Nanton J, Dhawan S, Pearce DJ, Feldman SR. Novel combination regimens: biologics and acitretin for the treatment of psoriasis - a case series. J Dermatol Treat. 2006;17:86–9. https://doi.org/10.1080/09546630500482928.
54. Gisondi P, Del Giglio M, Cotena C, Girolomoni G. Combining etanercept and acitretin in the therapy of chronic plaque psoriasis: a 24-week, randomized, controlled, investigator-blinded pilot trial. Br J Dermatol. 2008;158(6):1345–9. https://doi.org/10.1111/j.1365-2133.2008.08564.x.
55. Lee JH, Youn JI, Kim TY, Choi JH, Park CJ, Choe YB, et al. A multicenter, randomized, open-label pilot trial assessing the efficacy and safety of etanercept 50 mg twice weekly followed by etanercept 25 mg twice weekly, the combination of etanercept 25 mg twice weekly and acitretin, and acitretin alone in patients with moderate to severe psoriasis. BMC Dermatol. 2016;16(1):11. https://doi.org/10.1186/s12895-016-0048-z.
56. Smith EC, Riddle C, Menter MA, Lebwohl M. Combining systemic retinoids with biologic agents for moderate to severe psoriasis. Int J Dermatol. 2008;47(5):514–8. https://doi.org/10.1111/j.1365-4632.2008.03470.x.
57. Armstrong AW, Bagel J, Van Voorhees AS, Robertson AD, Yamauchi PS. Combining biologic therapies with other systemic treatments in psoriasis: evidence-based, best-practice recommendations from the Medical Board of the National Psoriasis Foundation. JAMA Dermatol. 2015;151(4):432–8. https://doi.org/10.1001/jamadermatol.2014.3456.
58. Polat Ekinci A, Bölük KN, Babuna Kobaner G. Secukinumab and acitretin as a combination therapy for three clinical forms of severe psoriasis in multidrug refractory patients: a case series of high efficacy and safety profile. Dermatol Ther. 2021;34(1):e14704. https://doi.org/10.1111/dth.14704.
59. Lee EJ, Shin MK, Kim NI. A clinical trial of combination therapy with etanercept and low dose cyclosporine for the treatment of refractory psoriasis. Ann Dermatol. 2010;22(2):138–42. https://doi.org/10.5021/ad.2010.22.2.138.
60. D'Angelo S, Cutro MS, Lubrano E, Leccese P, Mennillo GA, Ferrara N, et al. Combination therapy with ciclosporin and etanercept in patients with psoriatic arthritis. Ann Rheum Dis. 2010;69(5):934–5. https://doi.org/10.1136/ard.2009.119446.
61. Karanikolas GN, Koukli EM, Katsalira A, Arida A, Petrou D, Komninou E, et al. Adalimumab or cyclosporine as monotherapy and in combination in severe psoriatic arthritis: results from a prospective 12-month nonrandomized unblinded clinical trial. J Rheumatol. 2011;38(11):2466–74. https://doi.org/10.3899/jrheum.110242.
62. Yamauchi PS, Lowe NJ. Cessation of cyclosporine therapy by treatment with etanercept in patients with severe psoriasis. J Am Acad Dermatol. 2006;54(3 suppl 2):S135–8.
63. Cohen Barak E, Kerner M, Rozenman D, Ziv M. Combination therapy of cyclosporine and anti-tumor necrosis factor α in psoriasis: a case series of 10 patients. Dermatol Ther. 2015;28(3):126–30. https://doi.org/10.1111/dth.12196.
64. Gattu S, Wu J, Koo J. Can adalimumab make a smooth and easy transition from cyclosporine a reality? A case series of successful transitions. Psoriasis Forum. 2009;15a(2):33–5. https://doi.org/10.1177/247553030915a00206.
65. Ortiz A, Yamauchi PS. A treatment strategy for psoriasis: transitioning from systemic therapy to biologic agents. Skinmed. 2006;5:285–8. https://doi.org/10.1111/j.1540-9740.2006.05679.x.
66. Di Lernia V, Rossi F, De Fanti A. Etanercept combined with cyclosporine in a 6-year-old child with severe plaque psoriasis. J Dtsch Dermatol Ges. 2016;14(10):1042–3. https://doi.org/10.1111/ddg.13062.
67. Georgesen C, Wildman H, Wang X, Magro C. Pediatric pustular psoriasis responsive to cyclosporine bridged to etanercept: a treatment approach. Dermatol Online J. 2017;23(11). pii: 13030/qt9787b6c0.
68. Paul CF, Ho VC, McGeown C, Christophers E, Schmidtmann B, Guillaume JC, et al. Risk of malignancies in psoriasis patients treated with cyclosporine: a 5 y cohort study. J Invest Dermatol. 2003;120(2):211–6. https://doi.org/10.1046/j.1523-1747.2003.12040.x.
69. AbuHilal M, Walsh S, Shear N. Use of apremilast in combination with other therapies for treatment of chronic plaque psoriasis: a retrospective study. J Cutan Med Surg. 2016;20(4):313–6. https://doi.org/10.1177/1203475416631328.
70. Danesh MJ, Beroukhim K, Nguyen C, Levin E, Koo J. Apremilast and adalimumab: a novel combination therapy for recalcitrant psoriasis. Dermatol Online J. 2015;21(6). pii: 13030/qt5gf406zs.
71. Rothstein BE, McQuade B, Greb JE, Goldminz AM, Gottlieb AB. Apremilast and secukinumab combined therapy in a patient with recalcitrant plaque psoriasis. J Drugs Dermatol. 2016;15(5):648–9.
72. Sacchelli L, Patrizi A, Loi C, Bardazzi F. Combination therapy of apremilast and secukinumab in patients

with moderate-to-severe, recalcitrant plaque psoriasis. Clin Exp Dermatol. 2019;44(7):e243–4. https://doi.org/10.1111/ced.14000.
73. Cuchacovich R, Garcia-Valladares I, Espinoza LR. Combination biologic treatment of refractory psoriasis and psoriatic arthritis. J Rheumatol. 2012;39(1):187–93. https://doi.org/10.3899/jrheum.110295.
74. Babalola O, Lakdawala N, Strober BE. Combined biologic therapy for the treatment of psoriasis and psoriatic arthritis: a case report. JAAD Case Rep. 2015;1(1):3–4. https://doi.org/10.1016/j.jdcr.2014.09.002.
75. Gniadecki R, Bang B, Sand C. Combination of antitumour necrosis factor-alpha and anti-interleukin-12/23 antibodies in refractory psoriasis and psoriatic arthritis: a long-term case-series observational study. Br J Dermatol. 2016;174(5):1145–6. https://doi.org/10.1111/bjd.14270.
76. Torre KM, Payette MJ. Combination biologic therapy for the treatment of severe palmoplantar pustulosis. JAAD Case Rep. 2017;3(3):240–2. https://doi.org/10.1016/j.jdcr.2017.03.002.
77. Rathod D, Weinberg JM, Yamauchi PS. Successful treatment of refractory plaque-type psoriasis and psoriatic arthritis with guselkumab and adalimumab combination therapy: a case report. J Drugs Dermatol. 2019;18(4):394–6.
78. Thibodeaux Q, Ly K, Reddy V, Smith MP, Liao W. Dual biologic therapy for recalcitrant psoriasis and psoriatic arthritis. JAAD Case Rep. 2019;5(10):928–30. https://doi.org/10.1016/j.jdcr.2019.08.015.

7 Biologic Agents for the Treatment of Pediatric Psoriasis

Megan Mosca, Edward Hadeler, Tina Bhutani, and Kelly M. Cordoro

Psoriasis affects individuals of all ages with an estimated one-third of cases beginning in childhood [1]. The overall prevalence of psoriasis in children and adolescents ranges from 0.30% to 1.37% [2–4]. In addition to the skin manifestations, psoriasis in childhood is associated with several comorbid conditions, including obesity, hyperlipidemia, arthritis, anxiety, and depression [5–9]. Furthermore, children and adolescents with psoriasis, even in the presence of mild disease, experience impaired quality of life and stigmatization [10–12]. Undertreatment of psoriasis in childhood may drive poor psychosocial and health outcomes. The "psoriatic march," which is the hypothesized cascade from chronic uncontrolled inflammation to cardiovascular comorbidities in adulthood, is a compelling and biologically plausible rationale for adequately treating severe psoriasis in childhood [13, 14]. The recent increase in inclusion of pediatric patients in psoriasis clinical trials and the subsequent approval of targeted therapies by the FDA have leveled the therapeutic playing field for children by offering a balanced portfolio of treatment options with pediatric-specific data [14]. The rapidly growing body of evidence regarding the efficacy and safety, combined with the convenience of biologic therapy, has prompted increased utilization of these agents in the pediatric population. However, the use of biologics in children also presents challenges such as the need to deliver via injection and lack of access/insurance coverage, to name a few. Discussed below are the approved biologic agents, real-world clinical data, and practical recommendations for biologic initiation in pediatric psoriasis patients.

Clinical Trial Data

Currently, four agents, etanercept (ages 4 years and older), ustekinumab (6 years and older), ixekizumab (6 years and older), and secukinumab (6 years and older), are approved by the Food and Drug Administration (FDA) for the treatment of pediatric plaque psoriasis. In Europe, in addition to these four agents, adalimumab is also approved for use in children and adolescents aged 4 years and older. Several other biologics are approved for different conditions in the pediatric population and have been used off-label for the treatment of psoriasis. Clinical data on the FDA-approved biologics

M. Mosca (✉) · E. Hadeler
University of California, San Francisco, Department of Dermatology, Psoriasis and Skin Treatment Center, San Francisco, CA, USA
e-mail: ehadeler@med.miami.edu

T. Bhutani
Department of Dermatology, Psoriasis and Skin Treatment Center, University of California, San Francisco, San Francisco, CA, USA
e-mail: Tina.Bhutani@ucsf.edu

K. M. Cordoro
University of California San Francisco, Department of Dermatology, San Francisco, CA, USA
e-mail: Kelly.Cordoro@ucsf.edu

N. Brownstone et al. (eds.), *Biologic Therapy for Psoriasis*, Updates in Clinical Dermatology,
https://doi.org/10.1007/978-3-030-92938-1_7

for pediatric psoriasis is discussed below, and details of their indications in pediatric patients, clinical monitoring, dosing schedules, and adverse events as described on the FDA label are presented in Tables 7.1, 7.2, and 7.3, respectively.

TNF Inhibitors

Etanercept, a tumor necrosis factor (TNF)-α inhibitor, was the first biologic approved by the FDA for the treatment of plaque psoriasis in pediatric patients ages ≥4 years in 2016 [15, 16]. The randomized placebo-controlled phase III clinical trial of children ages 4–17 demonstrated that 57% of those treated with etanercept achieved Psoriasis Area and Severity Index (PASI) 75 (vs. 11% on placebo [$p < 0.001$]) [17]. By week 36, 68% of patients who continued on etanercept and 65% of patients who switched to etanercept after initial randomization to placebo achieved PASI 75. Longer-term data have demonstrated that etanercept is well tolerated and remains efficacious in pediatric patients for up to 264 weeks [18]. PASI 75 remained consistent between approximately 60 and 70% from weeks 96 through 264. The most commonly reported events were upper respiratory tract infections (37.6%), nasopharyngitis (26%), and headaches (21.5%). Between weeks 96 and 264, six patients withdrew from the study due to the following adverse events: Crohn's disease ($n = 2$), glomerulonephritis ($n = 1$), seventh nerve paralysis ($n = 1$), sinusitis ($n = 1$), and worsening of psoriasis ($n = 1$). Through week 264 only one serious adverse event (SAE) was determined to be related to etanercept treatment (cellulitis).

IL-12/23 Inhibitor

Ustekinumab, a human interleukin (IL)-12/23 antagonist, was FDA approved for moderate-to-severe plaque psoriasis in patients ages ≥12 years in 2017 and ages ≥6 years in 2020 [19–21]. The first randomized, placebo-controlled clinical trial evaluated ustekinumab at standard pediatric dosing (SD), ustekinumab at half-standard pediatric dosing (HSD), and placebo in patients ages 12–17 years with plaque psoriasis [22]. PASI 75 was achieved by 80.6% of patients receiving ustekinumab SD and 78.4% of patients receiving ustekinumab HSD (vs. 10.8% placebo [$p < 0.001$]). This response was well maintained throughout week 52 in all children receiving ustekinumab. Rates of adverse events were similar across all treatment groups through week 12 with the most commonly reported being nasopharyngitis (2.8% in SD, 13.5% in HSD, and 27.0% in placebo groups) and headache (8.3% in SD, 10.8% in HSD, and 5.4% in placebo groups). Through week 60, "infections and infestations" was the most commonly reported category of adverse event. The second phase III, open-label, single-arm clinical trial evaluated the standard dosing of ustekinumab in 44 patients ages 6–12 years [23, 24]. A total of 84% of patients achieved PASI 75 at week 12 and this response was well maintained through week 52. Nasopharyngitis (25%), pharyngitis (14%), and upper respiratory tract infection (14%) were the most common adverse events reported by study participants. No serious adverse events were deemed related to the study drug.

IL-17 Inhibitors

Ixekizumab, a humanized IL-17A antagonist, was approved by the FDA in 2020 for moderate-to-severe plaque psoriasis in pediatric patients ages ≥6 years [25, 26]. The randomized, placebo-controlled phase III trial demonstrated that ixekizumab was superior to placebo in the treatment of pediatric psoriasis patients ages 6–17 years [27]. PASI 75 was achieved by 89% in the ixekizumab group at week 12 (vs. 25% in the placebo group [$p < 0.001$]). This clinical response was well maintained with 90% of the ixekizumab group achieving PASI 75 at week 48. During the first 12 weeks, the most commonly reported adverse events included infections (129 patients [66%]) and injection site reactions (39 patients [20%]). Overall, two SAEs (Crohn's disease [$n = 2$]) were considered related to the study treatment.

Secukinumab, a human IL-17A antagonist, was the most recent biologic approved by the

Table 7.1 Data, dosage, and monitoring for TNF-α inhibitors

Drug[c]	Mechanism of action	Pediatric approvals	Baseline assessment	Monitoring[a]	Pediatric dosing schedules[b]	Contraindications/adverse effects	References
Etanercept (Enbrel)	Soluble fusion protein of TNF-α receptor and Fc portion of human IgG	FDA approved for polyarticular JIA in ages ≥2 and *plaque psoriasis in ages ≥4 (2016)* EMA approved for polyarthritis and extended oligoarthritis in ages ≥2, *plaque psoriasis in ages ≥6*, and psoriatic arthritis and enthesitis-related arthritis in ages ≥12	History and physical exam Severity assessment (objective and subjective) Assessment for comorbidities (individualized) Pretreatment testing for latent TB (PPD, T-Spot, or QuantiFERON Gold)	History and physical exam (every 3 months to 1 year) Latent TB testing once a year (PPD, T-Spot, or QuantiFERON Gold) Other labs/ evaluation as indicated	~0.8 mg/kg subcutaneous every week If >63 kg: 50 mg subcutaneous every week	Contraindicated in patients with active infection, sepsis, untreated hepatitis B, history of lymphoreticular malignancy, congestive heart failure, and multiple sclerosis Common adverse events include injection site reactions, upper respiratory tract infections, nasopharyngitis, and headaches	[15, 16, 33, 37–39]
Adalimumab (Humira)	Fully humanized monoclonal IgG antibody targeting TNF-α	FDA approved for JIA and uveitis in ages ≥2 and ≥10 kg, UC in ages ≥5, CD in ages ≥6, and HS in ages ≥12 EMA approved for polyarticular JIA and uveitis in ages ≥2, plaque psoriasis in ages ≥4, enthesitis-related arthritis and CD in ages ≥6	History and physical exam Severity assessment (objective and subjective) Assessment for comorbidities (individualized) Pretreatment testing for latent TB (PPD, T-Spot, or QuantiFERON Gold)	History and physical exam (every 3 months to 1 year) Latent TB testing once a year (PPD, T-Spot, or QuantiFERON Gold) Other labs/ evaluation as indicated	~ 24 mg/m^2 subcutaneous or 0.8 mg/kg (maximum 40 mg) at week 1 and 2, then every 2 weeks *(Per AAD-NPF guideline)*	Contraindicated in patients with active infection, sepsis, untreated hepatitis B, history of lymphoreticular malignancy, congestive heart failure, and multiple sclerosis Common adverse reactions include upper respiratory infections, sinusitis, injection site reactions, headache, and rash	[33, 37, 38, 40, 41]

(continued)

Table 7.1 (continued)

Drug[c]	Mechanism of action	Pediatric approvals	Baseline assessment	Monitoring[a]	Pediatric dosing schedules[b]	Contraindications/adverse effects	References
Infliximab (Remicade)	Chimeric monoclonal IgG antibody targeting TNF-α	FDA approved for CD and UC in ages ≥6 EMA approved for CD and UC in ages ≥6 [42]	History and physical exam Severity assessment (objective and subjective) Assessment for comorbidities (individualized) Pretreatment testing for latent TB (PPD, T-Spot, or QuantiFERON Gold)	History and physical exam (every 3 months to 1 year) Latent TB testing once a year (PPD, T-Spot, or QuantiFERON Gold) Other labs/evaluation as indicated	3.3–5 mg/kg intravenous at weeks 0, 2, and 6 and then every 7–8 weeks after *(Per FDA dosing for pediatric CD/UC and clinical guidelines)*	Contraindicated in patients with active infection, sepsis, untreated hepatitis B, history of lymphoreticular malignancy, congestive heart failure, and multiple sclerosis Common adverse reactions include upper respiratory infections, sinusitis, and pharyngitis, infusion-related reactions, headaches, and abdominal pain	[33, 37, 38, 42, 43]

Abbreviations: TNF tumor necrosis factor, *UC* ulcerative colitis, *CD* Crohn's disease, *JIA* juvenile idiopathic arthritis, *HS* hidradenitis suppurativa, *FDA* Food and Drug Administration, *EMA* European Medical Agency, *TB* tuberculosis, *PPD* purified protein derivative, *PASI* Psoriasis Area and Severity Index, *BSA* body surface area, *PGA* Physician Global Assessment, *AAD* American Academy of Dermatology, *NPF* National Psoriasis Foundation

[a]Additional laboratory monitoring, including complete blood count, liver functioning tests, HIV screening, hepatitis screening, etc., should be individualized based on the presence of comorbid disease and risk factors

[b]FDA-approved dosing for pediatric patients with plaque psoriasis unless otherwise stated

[c]Biologics that are FDA approved for pediatric plaque psoriasis are in italics

Table 7.2 Data, dosage, and monitoring for IL-17 inhibitors for the treatment of pediatric plaque psoriasis

Drug[c]	Mechanism of action	Pediatric approvals	Baseline assessment	Monitoring[a]	Pediatric dosing schedules[b]	Contraindications/adverse effects	References
Secukinumab (Consentyx)	Fully human IgG1 monoclonal antibody against IL-17	FDA approved for *moderate-to-severe plaque psoriasis in ages ≥6 (2021)* EMA approved for *plaque psoriasis in ages ≥6*	History and physical exam Severity assessment (objective and subjective) Assessment for comorbidities (individualized) Pretreatment testing for latent TB (PPD, T-Spot, or QuantiFERON Gold)	History and physical exam (every 3 months to 1 year) Other labs/evaluation as indicated	<50 kg: 75 mg subcutaneous at weeks 0, 1, 2, 3, and 4 and every 4 weeks after ≥50 kg: 150 mg subcutaneous at weeks 0, 1, 2, 3, and 4 and every 4 weeks after	Contraindicated in patients with active infection or active history/currently active inflammatory bowel disease Common adverse events include nasopharyngitis, headaches, pharyngitis, and rhinitis	[29, 33, 37, 38, 44, 45]
Ixekizumab (Taltz)	Humanized IgG4 monoclonal antibody against IL-17	FDA approved for *moderate-to-severe plaque psoriasis in ages ≥6 (2020)* EMA approved for *moderate-to-severe plaque psoriasis in ages ≥6 and ≥25 kg*	History and physical exam Severity assessment (objective and subjective) Assessment for comorbidities (individualized) Pretreatment testing for latent TB (PPD, T-Spot, or QuantiFERON Gold)	History and physical exam (every 3 months to 1 year) Other labs/evaluation as indicated	<25 kg: 40 mg subcutaneous at week 0 and then 20 mg every 4 weeks 25–50 kg: 80 mg subcutaneous at week 0 and then 40 mg every 4 weeks >50 kg: 160 mg subcutaneous at week 0 and then 80 mg every 4 weeks	Contraindicated in patients with active infection or active history/currently active inflammatory bowel disease Common adverse events include injection site reactions, upper respiratory tract infections, nausea, and tinea infections	[25, 26, 33, 37, 38, 46]

Abbreviations: FDA Food and Drug Administration, *EMA* European Medical Agency, *TB* tuberculosis, *PPD* purified protein derivative, *PASI* Psoriasis Area and Severity Index, *BSA* body surface area, *PGA* Physician Global Assessment

[a]Additional laboratory monitoring, including complete blood count, liver functioning tests, HIV screening, hepatitis screening, etc., should be individualized based on the presence of comorbid disease and risk factors

[b]FDA-approved dosing for pediatric patients with plaque psoriasis unless otherwise stated

[c]Biologics that are FDA approved for pediatric plaque psoriasis are in italics

Table 7.3 Data, dosage, and monitoring for IL-12/23 inhibitors

Drug[c]	Mechanism of action	Pediatric approvals	Baseline assessment	Monitoring[a]	Pediatric dosing schedules[b]	Contraindications/adverse effects	References
Ustekinumab (Stelara)	Fully human monoclonal antibody targeting the p40 subunit of IL-12 and IL-23	FDA approved for *plaque psoriasis in ages ≥ 6 (2020)* EMA approved for *plaque psoriasis in ages ≥6*	History and physical exam Severity assessment (objective and subjective) Assessment for comorbidities (individualized) Pretreatment testing for latent TB (PPD, T-Spot, or QuantiFERON Gold)	History and physical exam (every 3 months to 1 year) Other labs/evaluation as indicated	<60 kg: 0.75 mg/kg/dose subcutaneous at weeks 0 and 4 and every 12 weeks 60–100 kg: 45 mg subcutaneous at weeks 0 and 4 and every 12 weeks >100 kg: 90 mg subcutaneous, weeks 0 and 4 and then every 12 weeks	Contraindicated in patients with active infection, sepsis, untreated hepatitis B, and history of lymphoreticular malignancy Most common adverse events include nasopharyngitis, upper respiratory tract infection, headache, and fatigue	[19, 21, 33, 37, 38, 47]

Abbreviations: FDA Food and Drug Administration, *EMA* European Medical Agency, *TB* tuberculosis, *PPD* purified protein derivative, *PASI* Psoriasis Area and Severity Index, BSA body surface area, *PGA* Physician Global Assessment

[a]Additional laboratory monitoring, including complete blood count, liver functioning tests, HIV screening, hepatitis screening, etc., should be individualized based on the presence of comorbid disease and risk factors

[b]FDA-approved dosing for pediatric patients with plaque psoriasis unless otherwise stated

[c]Biologics that are FDA approved for pediatric plaque psoriasis are in italics

FDA in 2021 for treatment of moderate-to-severe plaque psoriasis in pediatric patients ages ≥6 years [28, 29]. The phase III randomized, controlled trial evaluating low-dose (LD) secukinumab (75 mg or 150 mg based on weight), high-dose (HD) secukinumab (75 mg, 150 mg, or 300 mg based on weight), etanercept 0.8 mg/kg, and placebo in children ages 6–18 with moderate-to-severe plaque psoriasis demonstrated that secukinumab was superior to placebo [30]. By week 12, PASI 75 was achieved by a significantly greater proportion of patients treated with LD secukinumab and HD secukinumab versus placebo (80% and 77.5% vs. 14.6%, respectively [$p < 0.0001$]). When compared to etanercept, LD secukinumab and HD secukinumab resulted in a numerically higher, but not statistically significant, percent of patients achieving PASI 75 at week 12 (80% and 77.5% vs. 63.4%, respectively). Clinical outcomes were maintained throughout the course of the study, and PASI 75 was achieved by 87.5% of patients treated with LD secukinumab, 87.5% treated with HD secukinumab, and 68.3% treated with etanercept at week 52. Overall, the incidence of adverse events (AEs) was similar in the LD secukinumab (80.4%), HD secukinumab (81%), and etanercept (82.9%) groups. The most commonly reported AEs in all secukinumab-treated patients were nasopharyngitis (29.8%), headaches (14.9%), pharyngitis (10.5%), and rhinitis (7.9%).

Real-World Usage Data

Real-world data on biologic therapies used for pediatric psoriasis have been published. One such study performed retrospectively in France evaluated the long-term safety, efficacy, and drug survival of adalimumab, etanercept, and ustekinumab in 134 pediatric patients with psoriasis [31]. This study demonstrated that ustekinumab had higher drug survival rates compared to etanercept and adalimumab ($p < 0.0001$). Additionally, drug survival rates were higher with ustekinumab and adalimumab than with etanercept in patients previously treated with other biologics ($p = 0.007$). Discontinuation of therapy due to primary inefficacy and loss of efficacy was more frequent with etanercept than with adalimumab or ustekinumab (etanercept, 15.9% and 34.9%; adalimumab, 3.7% and 9.1%; and ustekinumab, 2.9% and 0%, respectively). In total, eight SAEs were reported and only occurred in patients treated with TNF-α inhibitors. SAEs consisted of severe infections ($n = 3$), weight gain ($n = 2$), psoriasis flare ($n = 1$), and malaise ($n = 1$). Biologic therapy was discontinued in two children with associated weight gain, which did not improve after discontinuation of therapy, and one child with a psoriasis flare, which led to favorable outcome following discontinuation.

A second real-world retrospective cohort study of North American and European centers compared psoriasis severity and drug survival in pediatric psoriasis patients treated with biologics versus methotrexate [32]. While both biologics and methotrexate were associated with improvement of pediatric psoriasis, biologics were associated with greater efficacy. After potential confounders were controlled for, children on biologic therapy were significantly more likely to achieve Psoriasis Area Severity Index (PASI) 75 from baseline through 6 months when compared to those on methotrexate ($p < 0.001$). Patients on biologic agents also achieved greater reductions in PASI and Physician Global Assessment (PGA) scores throughout the 6 months of treatment when compared to methotrexate ($p < 0.05$). Biologics had longer drug survival than methotrexate ($p = 0.01$), but discontinuation of treatment due to lack of response was comparable in both treatment groups. However, suboptimal dosing of methotrexate and a short study duration may have underestimated the efficacy of methotrexate in this study. Furthermore, the results of the etanercept study in pediatric psoriasis patients were reported in the middle of the study period, which may have also impacted the drug survival of methotrexate.

While randomized controlled trials are the standard to assess efficacy and safety, these real-world cohorts can provide valuable information as well given the paucity of approved biologic agents and comparative treatment trials. Real-world studies can provide additional data for clinicians and families to consider during the shared decision-making process of treatment choice. On the other hand, it is also important to understand the overall utility of this data in the clinical context. Typically, these retrospective analyses offer an inferior level of evidence and suffer from inadequacies due to inaccurate and nonstandardized clinical record keeping. Furthermore, drug survival has many possible confounders not accounted for in these studies such as medication access and insurance coverage issues. Therefore, while real-world studies do provide some utility in an era where data on biologic treatment in pediatric patients is limited, the conclusions drawn from these studies should only be one of the many factors considered when selecting biologic therapy.

Currently, several other biologic therapies are being investigated for the treatment of plaque psoriasis in the pediatric population. Risankizumab (NCT04435600, NCT04862286), brodalumab (NCT04305327, NCT03240809), guselkumab (NCT03451851), bimekizumab (NCT04718896), tildrakizumab (NCT03997786), and certolizumab pegol (NCT04123795) all have ongoing clinical trials, but as of now are unapproved by the FDA for the treatment of pediatric plaque psoriasis.

Approach to Biologic Initiation

The baseline evaluation and laboratory work-up for pediatric patients with psoriasis when considering initiation of biologic treatment should be individualized to the specific clinical context [33]. All patients should undergo a comprehensive assessment including a history of present illness, past medical history, family history, current medications, and allergies and baseline clinical assessments to determine psoriasis type, distribution, severity, and comorbidities. Objective severity assessment tools include body surface area (BSA), Physician Global Assessment (PGA), and PASI. Joints should be examined to determine the presence of active arthritis. Blood pressure should be checked. Weight and height should be measured to calculate BMI. Pediatric patients and families should always be questioned about the impact of psoriasis on physical, social, emotional, and school functioning, as significant impairment of quality of life is a subjective index of severity [33]. Reassessment of disease severity to define response to therapy should be individualized to each patient but may occur every 3 months to 1 year.

The joint American Academy of Dermatology-National Psoriasis Foundation (AAD-NPF) guideline recommends baseline screening for latent tuberculosis (TB) with a purified protein derivative test (PPD), T-spot, or QuantiFERON Gold for children who are beginning biologic therapy [33]. If baseline screening for TB is positive, patients should be referred for further evaluation with an infectious disease specialist. Repeat yearly monitoring for latent TB is recommended for high-risk patients or patients who are being treated with a TNF-α inhibitor [33].

According to the current AAD-NPF guideline, no additional laboratory monitoring is required for otherwise healthy children on biologic therapy, but evaluations should be individualized to and evolve with each patient's unique clinical context and comorbid conditions [33]. Baseline labs and repeat monitoring also must account for monitoring for other systemic medications if combination therapy is used. Labs may include a complete blood count with differential, renal, and liver panels, lipids, and serologies for infection depending on the age of the patient and individual circumstances and risk factors. Hepatitis and HIV screening may be completed at baseline and repeated as indicated for children with risk factors [33].

Vaccinations require special consideration in pediatric patients who are beginning, or on, biologic therapy. Prior to initiation of therapy, a pediatric immunization history should be obtained, and live/live attenuated vaccinations ideally should be updated [14, 34]. If necessary, varicella and other viral immunity can be evaluated via serologic testing before starting treatment. A paucity of data exists on the safety and efficacy of live vaccines administered to pediatric patients receiving biologic therapy; therefore, guidelines vary on the procedure to follow if a patient requires a live immunization during treatment. Inactivated vaccines are generally considered safe to administer while on biologic therapy [34]. Antibody titers approximately 4–6 weeks after vaccine administration may be considered to confirm appropriate immunologic response; however most research has not demonstrated any reduction in antibody production [34]. Ultimately, decisions regarding vaccinations need to be determined based on the consideration of the severity of psoriasis and overall risks and circumstances for the patients. Overall, the goal is to ensure children stay up to date with health maintenance and obtain recommended vaccinations before, and during, biologic treatment. Families and other members of the patient's household should also be advised to update vaccinations prior to treatment initiation [33].

Special Considerations for Pediatric Psoriasis Patients with Biologics

Medical Decision-Making

There is no one size fits all approach when it comes to selecting a biologic therapy for a child with psoriasis. Choice depends on patient age, type of psoriasis, severity, speed of progression, comorbidities, and other factors. Establishing a strong therapeutic relationship with children and caregivers is essential when approaching the topic of any systemic psoriasis treatment. Engaging the family and patient in shared decision-making once the risks and benefits of not only the treatment options, but the risks of the disease itself, are discussed is important. It is clear from clinical trial data that biologic agents provide an opportunity for targeted high-efficacy treatment in pediatric patients, but they are not without risks and challenges. An in-depth discussion of the safety, efficacy, and logistics of available biologics with each family will allow informed decision-making and expectation management. Appropriate follow-up after initiation of biologic treatment provides the opportunity for patients and families to discuss questions or concerns.

Mode of Delivery

Treatment with injectable medications presents unique challenges in pediatric patients. The frequency of injections (weekly, bimonthly, etc.) may impact treatment choice. Regimens with a lower frequency of injections help decrease the burden placed on not only the child but also the caregivers. Additionally, a prefilled pen/autoinjector may be preferred over a classic syringe; however, the dosages available in autoinjectors will not always be suitable for pediatric patients depending on their weight. Etanercept (50 mg), adalimumab (80 mg and 40 mg), secukinumab (150 mg), and ixekizumab (80 mg) are all available as autoinjectors and may be used in pediatric patients if the dose is appropriate. When compared to syringes, prefilled pens were reported as significantly less painful by pediatric patients with juvenile idiopathic arthritis and were the preferred method of injection by caregivers [35].

Access

Another obstacle frequently faced by pediatric patients is the lack of insurance coverage and prohibitive costs for biologic treatments. In 2019, 41.4% of US children had public insurance, and 5.1% were uninsured, which suggests a large percentage of patients may have inadequate coverage for biologics [36]. Even with private insurance, coverage of biologics in pediatrics varies widely across different healthcare plans. Many plans require "step therapy," which is the requirement that the child is treated with a conventional systemic immune suppressive medication or phototherapy prior to the approval of a targeted biologic. These insurance barriers, which are not medically appropriate and based on cost alone, result in substantial undertreatment and increased health risks for a subset of pediatric patients. It is important to advocate for patients by appealing rejections and seeking peer-to-peer review with the physicians making authorization decisions within insurance companies.

Conclusion

Overall, growing evidence has shifted the landscape of treatment for children with psoriasis. Once an understudied, undertreated disease, we now have moved the treatment needle forward and should approach pediatric patients with psoriasis similarly to adults, but with special attention to the unique physical, psychological, and developmental needs of children of various ages. Drug selection and duration of therapy are individualized decisions that required consideration of multiple factors and shared decisions with patients and caregivers.

References

1. Raychaudhuri SP, Gross J. A comparative study of pediatric onset psoriasis with adult onset psoriasis. Pediatr Dermatol. 2000;17:174–8.
2. Wu JJ, Black MH, Smith N, Porter AH, Jacobsen SJ, Koebnick C. Low prevalence of psoriasis among children and adolescents in a large multiethnic cohort in southern California. J Am Acad Dermatol. 2011;65:957–64.
3. Augustin M, Glaeske G, Radtke MA, Christophers E, Reich K, Schäfer I. Epidemiology and comorbidity of psoriasis in children. Br J Dermatol. 2010;162:633–6.
4. Michalek IM, Loring B, John SM. A systematic review of worldwide epidemiology of psoriasis. J Eur Acad Dermatol Venereol. 2017;31:205–12.
5. Phan K, Lee G, Fischer G. Pediatric psoriasis and association with cardiovascular and metabolic comorbidities: systematic review and meta-analysis. Pediatr Dermatol. 2020;37:661–9.
6. Cho SI, Kim YE, Jo SJ. Association of metabolic comorbidities with pediatric psoriasis: a systematic review and meta-analysis. Ann Dermatol. 2021;33:203–13.
7. Paller AS, Schenfeld J, Accortt NA, Kricorian G. A retrospective cohort study to evaluate the development of comorbidities, including psychiatric comorbidities, among a pediatric psoriasis population. Pediatr Dermatol. 2019;36:290–7.
8. Kimball AB, Wu EQ, Guérin A, Yu AP, Tsaneva M, Gupta SR, Bao Y, Mulani PM. Risks of developing psychiatric disorders in pediatric patients with psoriasis. J Am Acad Dermatol. 2012;67:651–657.e1–2.
9. Brandon TG, Manos CK, Xiao R, Ogdie A, Weiss PF. Pediatric psoriatic arthritis: a population-based cohort study of risk factors for onset and subsequent risk of inflammatory comorbidities. J Psoriasis Psoriatic Arthritis. 2018;3:131–6.
10. Varni JW, Globe DR, Gandra SR, Harrison DJ, Hooper M, Baumgartner S. Health-related quality of life of pediatric patients with moderate to severe plaque psoriasis: comparisons to four common chronic diseases. Eur J Pediatr. 2012;171:485–92.
11. Salman A, Yucelten AD, Sarac E, Saricam MH, Perdahli-Fis N. Impact of psoriasis in the quality of life of children, adolescents and their families: a cross-sectional study. An Bras Dermatol. 2018;93:819–23.
12. Jager MEAD, Jong EMGJD, Evers AWM, Kerkhof PCMVD, Seyger MMB. The burden of childhood psoriasis. Pediatr Dermatol. 2011;28:736–7.
13. Boehncke W-H, Boehncke S, Tobin A-M, Kirby B. The 'psoriatic march': a concept of how severe psoriasis may drive cardiovascular comorbidity. Exp Dermatol. 2011;20:303–7.
14. Eichenfield LF, Paller AS, Tom WL, Sugarman J, Hebert AA, Friedlander SF, Siegfried E, Silverberg N, Cordoro KM. Pediatric psoriasis: evolving perspectives. Pediatr Dermatol. 2018;35:170–81.
15. FDA Approves Expanded Use Of ENBREL® (etanercept) to treat children with chronic moderate-to-severe plaque psoriasis. In: Amgen. https://www.amgen.com/newsroom/press-releases/2016/11/fda-approves-expanded-use-of-enbrel-etanercept-to-treat-children-with-chronic-moderatetosevere-plaque-psoriasis. Accessed 31 May 2021.
16. (2021) Highlights of prescribing information: Enbrel.
17. Paller AS, Siegfried EC, Langley RG, et al. Etanercept treatment for children and adolescents with plaque psoriasis. N Engl J Med. 2008;358:241–51.
18. Paller AS, Siegfried EC, Pariser DM, Rice KC, Trivedi M, Iles J, Collier DH, Kricorian G, Langley RG. Long-term safety and efficacy of etanercept in children and adolescents with plaque psoriasis. J Am Acad Dermatol. 2016;74:280–287.e1–3.
19. U.S. Food and Drug Administration Approves STELARA® (ustekinumab) for treatment of pediatric patients with moderate to severe plaque psoriasis. In: Janssen. https://www.janssen.com/us-food-and-drug-administration-approves-stelara-ustekinumab-treatment-pediatric-patients-moderate. Accessed 19 Nov 2020.
20. Janssen Announces U.S. FDA Approval of STELARA® (ustekinumab) for the Treatment of adolescents with moderate to severe plaque psoriasis | Johnson & Johnson. In: Content Lab U.S. https://www.jnj.com/media-center/press-releases/janssen-announces-us-fda-approval-of-stelara-ustekinumab-for-the-treatment-of-adolescents-with-moderate-to-severe-plaque-psoriasis. Accessed 13 July 2021.
21. (2020) Highlights of prescribing information: Stelara.
22. Landells I, Marano C, Hsu M-C, et al. Ustekinumab in adolescent patients age 12 to 17 years with moderate-to-severe plaque psoriasis: results of the randomized phase 3 CADMUS study. J Am Acad Dermatol. 2015;73:594–603.

23. Philipp S, Menter A, Nikkels AF, et al. Ustekinumab for the treatment of moderate-to-severe plaque psoriasis in paediatric patients (≥ 6 to < 12 years of age): efficacy, safety, pharmacokinetic and biomarker results from the open-label CADMUS Jr study. Br J Dermatol. 2020;183:664–72.
24. Philipp S, Menter A, Nikkels AF, et al. Results from the CADMUS Jr study: ustekinumab for treating plaque psoriasis in children. Br J Dermatol. 2020;183:e130.
25. Lilly's Taltz® (ixekizumab) Receives U.S. FDA approval for the treatment of pediatric patients with moderate to severe plaque psoriasis | Eli Lilly and Company. https://investor.lilly.com/news-releases/news-release-details/lillys-taltzr-ixekizumab-receives-us-fda-approval-treatment-1. Accessed 31 May 2021.
26. (2021) Highlights of prescribing information: Taltz.
27. Paller AS, Seyger MMB, Alejandro Magariños G, et al. Efficacy and safety of ixekizumab in a phase III, randomized, double-blind, placebo-controlled study in paediatric patients with moderate-to-severe plaque psoriasis (IXORA-PEDS). Br J Dermatol. 2020;183:231–41.
28. Novartis Cosentyx receives FDA approval for treatment of children and adolescents with moderate to severe plaque psoriasis. In: Novartis. https://www.novartis.com/news/media-releases/novartis-cosentyx-receives-fda-approval-treatment-children-and-adolescents-moderate-severe-plaque-psoriasis. Accessed 8 June 2021.
29. (2021) Highlights of prescribing information: Cosentyx.
30. Bodemer C, Kaszuba A, Kingo K, et al. Secukinumab demonstrates high efficacy and a favourable safety profile in paediatric patients with severe chronic plaque psoriasis: 52-week results from a phase 3 double-blind randomized, controlled trial. J Eur Acad Dermatol Venereol. 2021;35:938–47.
31. Phan C, Beauchet A, Burztejn A-C, et al. Biological treatments for paediatric psoriasis: a retrospective observational study on biological drug survival in daily practice in childhood psoriasis. J Eur Acad Dermatol Venereol. 2019;33:1984–92.
32. Bronckers IMGJ, Paller AS, West DP, et al. A comparison of psoriasis severity in pediatric patients treated with methotrexate vs biologic agents. JAMA Dermatol. 2020;156:384–92.
33. Menter A, Cordoro KM, Davis DMR, et al. Joint American Academy of Dermatology–National Psoriasis Foundation guidelines of care for the management and treatment of psoriasis in pediatric patients. J Am Acad Dermatol. 2020;82:161–201.
34. Munshi MA, Noe MH, Chiu YE, Streicher JL. Vaccines: considerations for pediatric dermatology patients on immunosuppressive agents. Pediatr Dermatol. https://doi.org/10.1111/pde.14631.
35. Roszkiewicz J, Swacha Z, Smolewska E. Prefilled pen versus prefilled syringe: a pilot study evaluating two different methods of methotrexate subcutaneous injection in patients with JIA. Pediatr Rheumatol Online J. 2020;18:64.
36. Cohen RA, Cha A, Martinez M, Terlizza E. Health insurance coverage: early release of estimates from the National Health Interview Survey, 2019. 2020; https://doi.org/10.1037/e565212009-001.
37. Brownstone ND, Hong J, Mosca M, Hadeler E, Liao W, Bhutani T, Koo J. Biologic treatments of psoriasis: an update for the clinician. Biologics. 2021;15:39–51.
38. Menter A, Strober BE, Kaplan DH, et al. Joint AAD-NPF guidelines of care for the management and treatment of psoriasis with biologics. J Am Acad Dermatol. 2019;80:1029–72.
39. European Medicines Agency (2021) European public assessment report: Enbrel.
40. European Medicines Agency (2021) European public assessment report: Humira.
41. (2021) Highlights of prescribing data: Humira.
42. European Medicines Agency (2020) European public assessment report: Remicade.
43. (2020) Highlights of prescribing information: Remicade.
44. European Medicines Agency (2021) European public assessment report: Cosentyx.
45. Novartis Cosentyx receives FDA approval for treatment of children and adolescents with moderate to severe plaque psoriasis. In: Novartis. https://www.novartis.com/news/media-releases/novartis-cosentyx-receives-fda-approval-treatment-children-and-adolescents-moderate-severe-plaque-psoriasis. Accessed 8 Jun 2021.
46. European Medicines Agency (2021) European public assessment report: Taltz.
47. European Medicines Agency (2020) European public assessment report overview: Stelara.

8 Special Site Psoriasis

Julie Hong, Megan Mosca, Edward Hadeler, Marwa Hakimi, and Wilson Liao

Nail Psoriasis: Efficacy and Safety of Biologic Treatments

Nail psoriasis can occur in about 10–82% of patients with plaque psoriasis and can cause a disproportionate amount of impairment on health-related quality of life, despite its small portion of the body surface area [1]. Clinical features of nail psoriasis can involve pitting, crumbling, oil drop discoloration, splinter hemorrhages, and loosening of the nail plates. Psoriasis in the nail can be difficult to treat and commonly relapses. Therapies should consider the severity of the nail disease, body surface area of skin involvement, presence of psoriatic arthritis, and impairment of quality of life. Systemic therapies are not typically recommended for the treatment of psoriasis that is isolated in the nails, unless the nail involvement causes functional impairment and significantly affects quality of life [2]. Systemic therapies, such as biologics, are often considered when patients have concomitant skin involvement.

J. Hong (✉)
University of California, San Francisco, Department of Dermatology, Psoriasis and Skin Treatment Center, San Francisco, CA, USA
e-mail: Julie.Hong2@ucsf.edu

M. Mosca
University of Nevada, Reno School of Medicine, Reno, NV, USA

E. Hadeler
University of Miami Leonard M. Miller School of Medicine, Miami, FL, USA

M. Hakimi · W. Liao
University of California, San Francisco, Department of Dermatology, Psoriasis and Skin Treatment Center, San Francisco, CA, USA

TNF-α Inhibitors

Adalimumab

A phase II randomized clinical trial evaluated the efficacy and safety of adalimumab for the treatment of nail psoriasis [3]. Patients with moderate-to-severe fingernail psoriasis and moderate-to-severe plaque psoriasis were randomized 1:1 to either adalimumab 40 mg every other week or placebo. 188 patients completed 26 weeks of treatment, and 46.6% of patients achieved Nail Psoriasis Severity Index (NAPSI-75) response or 75% reduction from baseline in NAPSI score at Week 26 compared to 3.4% of placebo patients [$p < 0.001$].

Etanercept

In a randomized controlled trial, 60 patients were randomized to receive adalimumab, etanercept, or infliximab for 24 weeks to treat nail psoriasis [4]. Etanercept was administered at a dose of 50 mg two times per week for 12 weeks and then 25 mg two times per week for 12 weeks for a total of 24 weeks of treatment. In the etanercept group, the mean NAPSI decreased from 34.8 at baseline to 10.6 at Week 24 ($p < 0.0016$). Among

N. Brownstone et al. (eds.), *Biologic Therapy for Psoriasis*, Updates in Clinical Dermatology,
https://doi.org/10.1007/978-3-030-92938-1_8

the three biologic therapies, the infliximab group showed significant improvement in NAPSI at Week 12, but both etanercept and adalimumab showed great improvement at Week 24.

Infliximab

A 50-week phase III study randomized patients with moderate-to-severe psoriasis to receive either infliximab or placebo, with placebo crossover to infliximab at Week 24 [5]. In 305 of 373 (81.8%) patients who had baseline nail psoriasis, 6.9%, 26.2%, and 44.7% in the infliximab group had nail disease clearance at weeks 10, 24, and 50, respectively, compared to 5.1% in the placebo group at Week 24 [$p < 0.001$]. Mean percent improvement in the NAPSI response was also superior in the infliximab group compared to the placebo group at Week 10 (26.8% vs. −7.7%) and Week 24 (57.2% vs. −4.1%) [$p < 0.001$].

IL-12/23 Inhibitor

Ustekinumab

The efficacy of ustekinumab in treating moderate-to-severe psoriasis was assessed in the PHOENIX 1 trial [6]. Patients were randomized to receive ustekinumab 45 mg, ustekinumab 90 mg, or placebo at weeks 0 and 4, with placebo crossover to ustekinumab at weeks 12 and 16. 545 of 766 (71.1%) patients had nail psoriasis, and the ustekinumab 45 mg group and 90 mg group showed 46.5% and 48.7% improvement, respectively, from baseline NAPSI score at Week 12. Patients continued to show improvement at Week 24 for both treatment groups (46.5% in ustekinumab 45 mg and 48.7% in ustekinumab 90 mg).

IL-17 Inhibitor

Brodalumab

The efficacy of brodalumab for the treatment of nail psoriasis was evaluated in three phase III trials (AMAGINE-2/-3) [7]. Nail clearance was measured for patients who received either brodalumab 210 mg every 2 weeks or ustekinumab through 52 weeks of treatment period. Patients who received brodalumab achieved greater improvement of mean NAPSI score at Week 12 (43.7% vs. 31.8%), Week 24 (76.9% vs. 58.9%), Week 36 (82.4% vs. 69.0%), and Week 52 (83.1% vs. 75.0%). Patients receiving brodalumab also achieved significantly greater complete clearance of nail psoriasis and higher mean percent improvement from baseline NAPSI compared to patients who received ustekinumab.

Ixekizumab

A phase III, double-blind, randomized controlled trial evaluated the effect of ixekizumab on nail psoriasis (UNCOVER-3) [8]. Patients with moderate-to-severe psoriasis were randomized to receive ixekizumab 80 mg every 2 weeks (Q2W) or 4 weeks (Q4W) after a 160 mg loading dose, etanercept 50 mg, or placebo through Week 60. At Week 12, patients in the ixekizumab group achieved greater mean NAPSI improvement (36.7% in Q4W and 35.2% in Q2W) compared to etanercept (20.0%) and placebo (−34.3%). Additionally, 19.7% in the ixekizumab Q4W group and 17.5% in the ixekizumab Q2W group achieved complete resolution of nail psoriasis compared to 10.2% etanercept and 4.3% placebo [$p < 0.05$].

Similarly, the IXORA-R trial compared the efficacy of ixekizumab and guselkumab [9]. Patients with moderate-to-severe-plaque psoriasis were randomized to receive ixekizumab 80 mg or guselkumab 100 mg. The ixekizumab group achieved PASI 100 as early as Week 2 and showed completely clear nails by Week 24 compared to the guselkumab group (52.0% vs. 31.0% [$p < 0.007$]). Patients on ixekizumab also demonstrated greater improvement in Dermatology Life Quality Index (DLQI) of 0 or 1 and lower itch rating [$p < 0.05$].

Secukinumab

In the TRANSFIGURE trial, patients with moderate-to-severe plaque and nail psoriasis were randomized to secukinumab 150 mg and secukinumab 300 mg [10]. At Week 16, both doses of secukinumab showed superior improvement in NAPSI score (45.3% secukinumab 300 mg and 37.9% secukinumab 150 mg) compared to placebo (10.8%) [$p < 0.001$]. Patients treated with secukinumab also experienced improvement in quality of life [$p < 0.001$]. The efficacy of secukinumab treatment was maintained up to Week 132 for both doses (73.3% secukinumab 300 mg and 63.6% secukinumab 150 mg) compared to placebo.

IL-23 Inhibitors

Guselkumab

A post hoc data analysis of VOYAGE 1 and VOYAGE 2, which are two double-blinded, randomized controlled trials, assessed the effect of guselkumab on nail psoriasis [11]. Patients were randomized to guselkumab 100 mg, adalimumab, or placebo crossover to guselkumab 100 mg at Week 16. At Week 0, 928/1829 (50.7%) patients had a score of 2 or higher for Fingernail Physician Global Assessment (f-PGA). At Week 16, 46.7% in the guselkumab group achieved f-PGA of 0.1 compared to 15.2% in the placebo group [$p < 0.001$]. There was no statistical difference at Week 24 (64% vs. 60% [$p < 0.11$]).

Summary

In treating nail psoriasis, biologic agents have shown superior long-term efficacy compared to topical treatment and other systemic therapies. IL-17 inhibitors (e.g., brodalumab and ixekizumab) have shown superior short-term efficacy compared to IL-12/23 inhibitors (e.g., ustekinumab), IL-23 inhibitors (e.g., guselkumab), and TNF-α inhibitors (e.g., etanercept). The long-term nail efficacy of IL-17 inhibitors is similar to that of TNF-α inhibitors. IL-23 inhibitors (e.g., guselkumab) have similar nail efficacy to certain TNF-a inhibitors (e.g., adalimumab).

Scalp Psoriasis: Efficacy and Safety of Biologic Treatments

Involvement of the scalp occurs in approximately 80% of patients with plaque psoriasis, making it one of the most commonly affected regions of the body [12]. Scalp psoriasis can be difficult to treat due to the location, poor accessibility, and lack of cosmetic appeal of various topical treatment options. Because of this, scalp psoriasis can lead to significant psychological and social impairment [13]. Optimizing therapy is critical to improve patient outcomes, satisfaction, and quality of life. Recent research has demonstrated that biologics are highly effective in the treatment of scalp psoriasis and may be a suitable first-line option for patients with scalp plaques plus whole-body psoriasis [14].

TNF-α Inhibitors

Etanercept

Etanercept was one of the first biologics shown to be effective for the treatment of moderate-to-severe scalp psoriasis. In 2012, a randomized, double-blind, placebo-controlled study compared etanercept 50 mg twice weekly for 12 weeks followed by etanercept 50 mg once weekly (group A) for 12 weeks and placebo for 12 weeks followed by etanercept 50 mg twice weekly for 12 weeks (group B). At Week 12, etanercept was superior to placebo in Psoriasis Scalp Severity Index (PSSI) 75 rates (etanercept: 86% vs placebo: 11% [$p < 0.0001$]) [15]. By Week 24, both group A and group B achieved mean PSSI improvements of 90.6% and 79.1%, respectively. Rates of adverse events were similar between etanercept and placebo treatment groups. Head-to-head studies of etanercept compared with other biologics for the treatment of scalp psoriasis are discussed below.

Adalimumab

Adalimumab has demonstrated good efficacy for the treatment of scalp psoriasis in two clinical trials [16, 17]. In a post hoc analysis of the randomized, controlled, phase III study, BELIEVE, patients were randomized to receive adalimumab plus topical calcipotriol and betamethasone or adalimumab plus vehicle [17]. At baseline, patients had a mean PSSI score of 17.9 ± 14.1; however, after 16 weeks of therapy with adalimumab, 77.8% of patients achieved a PSSI score of ≤4. The second multicenter, single-arm prospective clinical trial observed patients being treated with adalimumab for 12 months [16]. At baseline, patients had a mean PSSI of 26.8; however, after 1 year of treatment with adalimumab the mean PSSI improved by 94.8% to 1.2. By the end of year 1, 71.7% of patients had complete clearance of the scalp (PSSI score of 0). Rates of adverse events were similar to prior studies with adalimumab treatment.

IL-17 Inhibitors

Brodalumab

Brodalumab was superior compared to placebo for the treatment of scalp psoriasis in two clinical trials [7, 18]. In a randomized, double-blind, placebo-controlled, phase II trial randomized patients to receive brodalumab 70 mg, 140 mg, 210 mg, or placebo [7]. By Week 12, brodalumab 140 mg and 210 mg led to significantly greater reductions in PSSI from baseline compared to placebo (140 mg: −73.8%, 210 mg: −94.5% vs placebo: −12.6% [$p < 0.001$]). In the post hoc analysis of the randomized, double-blind, placebo-controlled, phase III study, AMAGINE-1, patients receiving brodalumab achieved significantly higher rates of PSSI 75 and PSSI 100 at Week 12 compared to placebo (PSSI 75, brodalumab: 89.0% vs placebo: 9.5%; PSSI 100, brodalumab 63.1% vs 3.2% [$p < 0.001$]) [18]. Brodalumab was also superior to placebo in achieving a greater percent improvement from baseline PSSI (92.8% vs 14.4%, respectively [$p < 0.001$]). The most common adverse events across both clinical trials with brodalumab include nasopharyngitis, diarrhea, and upper respiratory tract infections.

Secukinumab

Secukinumab demonstrated superiority when compared to placebo and good efficacy when evaluated in a real-world setting [19–21]. In the randomized, double-blind, placebo-controlled phase III clinical trial, patients with moderate-to-severe scalp psoriasis were randomized to receive secukinumab 300 mg or placebo for 20 weeks [19]. At Week 12, secukinumab achieved significantly higher rates of PSSI 90 than placebo (52.9% vs 2.0%, respectively [$p < 0.001$]). Secukinumab treatment was also superior compared to placebo in achieving complete clearance of the scalp by Week 12 (35.3% vs 0% [$p < 0.001$]). In a randomized, double-blind, placebo-controlled study, secukinumab achieved greater improvements in patient-reported pain (−1.98 vs 0.61), itching (−4.07 vs −0.04), scaling (−5.76 vs −0.95), and dermatitis-related quality of life (Scalpdex total: −39.62 vs −7.91) when compared to placebo at Week 12 ($p < 0.001$ for all) [20]. A two-year observational study evaluating the real-world data of secukinumab for the treatment of scalp psoriasis in 76 patients demonstrated that scalp physician global assessment (sPGA) rate was improved by 98.7% following 16 weeks of treatment [21]. Overall, the safety profile of secukinumab was consistent with previous clinical trials. The most common adverse events were nasopharyngitis, upper respiratory tract infections, contact dermatitis, and cough. Secukinumab also includes efficacy data of scalp psoriasis in the FDA label.

Ixekizumab

Overall, five clinical trials evaluating ixekizumab for the treatment of scalp psoriasis demonstrated that ixekizumab has good and sustained efficacy [22–24]. A post hoc analysis of a randomized, placebo-controlled phase II clinical trial randomized patients to receive ixekizumab 10, 25, 75, or 150 mg or placebo [22]. At Week 20, patients treated with ixekizumab 25 mg, 75 mg, and 150 mg achieved significantly higher mean percent reductions from baseline PSSI compared to placebo (75.3%, 83.7%, 82.2%, vs 18.8%, respectively $p < 0.01$). By Week 48, 78% of patients treated with ixekizumab achieved complete clearance of their scalp psoriasis.

In three phase III clinical trials, UNCOVER-1, UNCOVER-2, and UNCOVER-3, ixekizumab was shown to be superior to etanercept and placebo [23]. In UNCOVER-1, ixekizumab 80 mg at 2-week intervals or 4-week intervals was compared to placebo; however, UNCOVER-2/3 also compared ixekizumab head-to-head with etanercept. Pooled data from all three studies at Week 12 showed that ixekizumab every 2 weeks and ixekizumab every 4 weeks were superior to etanercept and placebo at achieving PSSI 90 and PSSI 100 (ixe every 2 wks: 81.7% and 74.6%; ixe every 4 wks: 75.6% and 68.9%; etanercept: 55.5% and 48.1%; placebo: 7.6% and 6.7% [$p < 0.001$ for all]).

The long-term extension of UNCOVER-3 demonstrated that PSSI 90 and PSSI 100 were maintained until Week 60 in patients initially treated with the ixekizumab 2-week dosing who were switched to 4-week dosing schedules, as well as patients continued on the ixekizumab 4-week dosing schedule. Another randomized, phase III clinical study compare three dosing schedules of ixekizumab: 80 mg every 2 weeks, 80 mg every 4 weeks, and 4- to 2-week interval dose adjustment groups [24]. At Week 52, complete clearance (PSSI score of 0) was achieved by 76.9% of patients with 2-week dosing, 70.3% of patients with the 4-week dosing, and 72.6% of patients with the 4- to 2-week dosing, respectively. Adverse events were similar across treatment arms in all studies, and the most common adverse events were upper respiratory tract infections, nasopharyngitis, and injection site reaction.

IL-23 Inhibitors

Guselkumab

A post hoc data analysis from data collected from VOYAGE 1 and VOYAGE 2 studied the efficacy of guselkumab in the treatment of scalp psoriasis [11]. Greater percentage of patients in the guselkumab group achieved scalp-specific IGA score of 0 or 1 at Week 24 compared to those in the adalimumab group (85% vs. 68.5% [$p < 0.001$]). Greater percentage of patients in the guselkumab group also achieved complete clearance of scalp psoriasis compared to the adalimumab group (69.9% vs. 56.3%).

Risankizumab

In a phase II trial, the efficacy of risankizumab was compared to that of ustekinumab for the treatment of scalp psoriasis [25]. At Week 12, the risankizumab 90 mg group and risankizumab 180 mg group showed 90% and 94% improvement in the mean PSSI score, respectively, compared to 82% improvement in the ustekinumab group. The mean percent PSSI change from baseline was maintained above 80% in patients receiving both doses of risankizumab.

Summary

Overall, patients who present with scalp psoriasis and moderate-to-severe plaque psoriasis should be considered for biologic therapy. Guselkumab and secukinumab present with clinical trial data on their FDA drug label, which could affect how insurance cover the costs of these drugs.

Genital/Inverse Psoriasis: Efficacy and Safety of Biologic Treatments

Psoriasis is one of the most common skin diseases that affects the genitalia with about 63% of patients with psoriasis developing genital lesions [26]. Genital psoriasis may present with atypical features of psoriasis and may cause great amount of emotional distress and sexual dysfunctions, which lead to poor quality of life. Patients with severe and recalcitrant genital psoriasis are treated with biologic therapies. A recent consensus statement by the International Psoriasis Council was developed to consider patients with genital psoriasis with mild symptoms of plaque psoriasis to warrant receiving systemic therapies, including biologics [27].

IL-17 Inhibitors

Ixekizumab

Ixekizumab is the only biologic therapy that has been studied in clinical trials for the treatment of genital psoriasis. A phase II clinical trial studied the long-term efficacy of ixekizumab through 52 weeks [28]. Patients received either ixekizumab 80 mg or placebo until Week 12, with a placebo crossover to ixekizumab 80 mg through Week 52. Greater percentage of patients in the ixekizumab group achieved static Physician's Global Assessment of Genitalia (sPGA-G) score of 0 or 1 compared to placebo at Week 12 (73% vs. 8% [$p < 0.001$]). 79% of patients in the placebo crossover group also showed rapid improvement in sPGA-G 0/1 at Week 52.

Other Biologics

Adalimumab and ustekinumab have been shown to treat inverse psoriasis in two separate case studies. One patient was treated with adalimumab 40 mg every 2 weeks for 90 days and showed complete regression of genital psoriasis [29]. One patient was treated with ustekinumab 45 mg every 4 weeks for the first month and then 45 mg every 12 weeks thereafter [30]. The patient paused the ustekinumab treatment after the first injection due to an adverse event of external otitis with tympanic perforation, but was subsequently restarted on ustekinumab 3 months later and achieved improvements in pruritus, erythema, and quality of life.

Summary

Psoriasis biologics, specifically ixekizumab, are recommended for patients with genital psoriasis. Currently, ixekizumab is the only biologic therapy that presents with clinical trial data on genital psoriasis in its FDA label. There are several papers that have demonstrated significant improvement in physical symptoms and quality of life in patients treated with ixekizumab.

Palmoplantar Psoriasis: Efficacy and Safety of Biologic Treatments

Palmoplantar psoriasis presents with thick, hyperkeratotic plaques and pustular features in the palms and soles and can affect 11–39% of patients with plaque psoriasis on other parts of the body. Clinical trials have shown that biologics are effective and well-tolerated in patients with both subtypes of palmoplantar psoriasis, hyperkeratotic and pustular.

TNF-α Inhibitors

Adalimumab

In a double-blinded, randomized placebo-controlled trial, 72 patients with hyperkeratotic palmoplantar psoriasis were randomized 2:1 to adalimumab 80 mg at Week 0 and 40 mg every 2 weeks thereafter and placebo through 16 weeks [31]. 30.6% patients who were treated with adalimumab achieved Physician Global Assessment of the hand and foot (hfPGA) score of 0 or 1 at Week 16 compared to only 4.3% of patients who were treated with placebo [$p < 0.01$].

Infliximab

The efficacy of infliximab was studied in a double-blinded randomized placebo-controlled trial in patients with hyperkeratotic palmoplantar psoriasis [32]. After 14 weeks of treatment, greater percentage of patients in the infliximab group achieved the modified Palmoplantar Pustulosis Area and Severity Index (m-PPPASI) 50 and 75 (66.7% and 33.3%, respectively) compared to 8.3% in the placebo group ($p = 0.009$ and 0.317, respectively). There was a 50.3% reduction in the mean surface area affected in the treatment group versus 14.9% increase in surface area in the placebo group.

IL-23 Inhibitors

Guselkumab

In VOYAGE 1, a phase III randomized clinical trial, guselkumab showed greater improvement in reducing the symptoms of hyperkeratotic palmoplantar psoriasis compared to adalimumab and placebo [33]. At Week 16, 73.3% patients receiving guselkumab 100 mg achieved IGA 0/1 compared to 55.8% in the adalimumab group and 14.0% in the placebo group. The efficacy was maintained at Week 24 for guselkumab (78.9%) versus adalimumab (56.8%) and at Week 48 (75.6% vs. 62.1%).

IL-17 Inhibitors

Ixekizumab

The efficacy of Ixekizumab in treating palmoplantar psoriasis was analyzed in the UNCOVER randomized clinical trial [34]. Patients were randomized to receive ixekizumab (160 mg at Week 0, 80 mg every 2 or 4 weeks) or etanercept (50 mg twice weekly) for up to 60 weeks. At Week 12, improvement in the PPASI score was greater in the ixekizumab group (80.0%) compared to the etanercept (53.0%) and the placebo (28.1%) groups [$p < 0.05$].

Secukinumab

In the GESTURE randomized clinical trial, 137 patients were randomized to receive secukinumab 300 mg, 150 mg, or placebo for the treatment of palmoplantar psoriasis [35]. Significantly greater percentage in both dosage group of secukinumab achieved PPIGA 0/1 (33.3% in 300 mg regimen, 22.1% in 150 mg regimen) compared to 1.5% of the placebo group [$p < 0.001$ and 0.002, respectively]. DLQI 0/1 was achieved in 26.6% of the secukinumab 300 mg group and 16.9% of the secukinumab 150 mg group compared to 1.5% in the placebo group [$p < 0.0001$ and 0.0005, respectively]. Another randomized controlled trial showed that patients who received secukinumab 150 mg at weeks 0, 1, 2, and 4 achieved an IGA response versus the placebo group (54.3% vs. 19.2% [$p < 0.0005$]) [36].

Discussion

Studies have shown that biologic therapies are effective and safe for the treatment of palmoplantar psoriasis. Adalimumab, guselkumab, ixekizumab, and secukinumab have shown greater than 80% in treatment efficacy for hyperkeratotic palmoplantar psoriasis. Infliximab has moderate efficacy in the treatment of pustular psoriasis.

References

1. Bardazzi F, Lambertini M, Chessa MA, Magnano M, Patrizi A, Piraccini BM. Nail involvement as a negative prognostic factor in biological therapy for psoriasis: a retrospective study. J Eur Acad Dermatol Venereol. 2017;31(5):843–6. https://doi.org/10.1111/jdv.13979.
2. Sánchez-Regaña M, Sola-Ortigosa J, Alsina-Gibert M, Vidal-Fernández M, Umbert-Millet P. Nail psoriasis: a retrospective study on the effectiveness of systemic treatments (classical and biological therapy): nail psoriasis, effectiveness of systemic treatments. J Eur Acad Dermatol Venereol. 2011;25(5):579–86. https://doi.org/10.1111/j.1468-3083.2010.03938.x.
3. Elewski BE, Okun MM, Papp K, et al. Adalimumab for nail psoriasis: efficacy and safety from the first 26 weeks of a phase 3, randomized, placebo-controlled trial. J Am Acad Dermatol. 2018;78(1):90–99.e1. https://doi.org/10.1016/j.jaad.2017.08.029.
4. Saraceno R, Pietroleonardo L, Mazzotta A, Zangrilli A, Bianchi L, Chimenti S. TNF-α antagonists and nail psoriasis: an open, 24-week, prospective cohort study in adult patients with psoriasis. Expert Opin Biol Ther. 2013;13(4):469–73. https://doi.org/10.1517/14712598.2013.736960.
5. Rich P, Griffiths CEM, Reich K, et al. Baseline nail disease in patients with moderate to severe psoriasis and response to treatment with infliximab during 1 year. J Am Acad Dermatol. 2008;58(2):224–31. https://doi.org/10.1016/j.jaad.2007.07.042.
6. Rich P, Bourcier M, Sofen H, et al. Ustekinumab improves nail disease in patients with moderate-to-severe psoriasis: results from PHOENIX 1. Br J Dermatol. 2014;170(2):398–407. https://doi.org/10.1111/bjd.12632.
7. Elewski B, Rich P, Lain E, Soung J, Lewitt GM, Jacobson A. Efficacy of brodalumab in the treatment of scalp and nail psoriasis: results from three phase 3

trials. J Dermatolog Treat. 2020:1–5. https://doi.org/10.1080/09546634.2020.1749546.
8. van de Kerkhof P, Guenther L, Gottlieb AB, et al. Ixekizumab treatment improves fingernail psoriasis in patients with moderate-to-severe psoriasis: results from the randomized, controlled and open-label phases of UNCOVER-3. J Eur Acad Dermatol Venereol. 2017;31(3):477–82. https://doi.org/10.1111/jdv.14033.
9. Blauvelt A, Leonardi C, Elewski B, et al. A head-to-head comparison of ixekizumab vs. guselkumab in patients with moderate-to-severe plaque psoriasis: 24-week efficacy and safety results from a randomized, double-blinded trial. Br J Dermatol. 2021;184(6):1047–58. https://doi.org/10.1111/bjd.19509.
10. Reich K, Sullivan J, Arenberger P, et al. Effect of secukinumab on the clinical activity and disease burden of nail psoriasis: 32-week results from the randomized placebo-controlled TRANSFIGURE trial. Br J Dermatol. 2019;181(5):954–66. https://doi.org/10.1111/bjd.17351.
11. Foley P, Gordon K, Griffiths CEM, et al. Efficacy of guselkumab compared with adalimumab and placebo for psoriasis in specific body regions: a secondary analysis of 2 randomized clinical trials. JAMA Dermatol. 2018;154(6):676–83. https://doi.org/10.1001/jamadermatol.2018.0793.
12. Chan CS, Van Voorhees AS, Lebwohl MG, et al. Treatment of severe scalp psoriasis: from the Medical Board of the National Psoriasis Foundation. J Am Acad Dermatol. 2009;60(6):962–71. https://doi.org/10.1016/j.jaad.2008.11.890.
13. Koo J, Marangell LB, Nakamura M, et al. Depression and suicidality in psoriasis: review of the literature including the cytokine theory of depression. J Eur Acad Dermatol Venereol. 2017;31(12):1999–2009. https://doi.org/10.1111/jdv.14460.
14. Mosca M, Hong J, Hadeler E, Brownstone N, Bhutani T, Liao W. Scalp psoriasis: a literature review of effective therapies and updated recommendations for practical management. Dermatol Ther (Heidelb). 2021;11(3):769–97. https://doi.org/10.1007/s13555-021-00521-z.
15. Bagel J, Lynde C, Tyring S, Kricorian G, Shi Y, Klekotka P. Moderate to severe plaque psoriasis with scalp involvement: a randomized, double-blind, placebo-controlled study of etanercept. J Am Acad Dermatol. 2012;67(1):86–92. https://doi.org/10.1016/j.jaad.2011.07.034.
16. Khobzey K, Liskova I, Szegedi A, et al. Effectiveness of adalimumab in the treatment of scalp and nail affection in patients with moderate to severe plaque psoriasis in routine clinical practice. Acta Dermatovenerol Alp Pannonica Adriat. 2017;26(1):11–4. https://doi.org/10.15570/actaapa.2017.3.
17. Thaçi D, Unnebrink K, Sundaram M, Sood S, Yamaguchi Y. Adalimumab for the treatment of moderate to severe psoriasis: subanalysis of effects on scalp and nails in the BELIEVE study. J Eur Acad Dermatol Venereol. 2015;29(2):353–60. https://doi.org/10.1111/jdv.12553.
18. Nakagawa H, Niiro H, Ootaki K. Japanese brodalumab study group. Brodalumab, a human anti-interleukin-17-receptor antibody in the treatment of Japanese patients with moderate-to-severe plaque psoriasis: efficacy and safety results from a phase II randomized controlled study. J Dermatol Sci. 2016;81(1):44–52. https://doi.org/10.1016/j.jdermsci.2015.10.009.
19. Bagel J, Duffin KC, Moore A, et al. The effect of secukinumab on moderate-to-severe scalp psoriasis: results of a 24-week, randomized, double-blind, placebo-controlled phase 3b study. J Am Acad Dermatol. 2017;77(4):667–74. https://doi.org/10.1016/j.jaad.2017.05.033.
20. Feldman SR, Green L, Kimball AB, et al. Secukinumab improves scalp pain, itching, scaling and quality of life in patients with moderate-to-severe scalp psoriasis. J Dermatolog Treat. 2017;28(8):716–21. https://doi.org/10.1080/09546634.2017.1329502.
21. Rompoti N, Katsimbri P, Kokkalis G, et al. Real world data from the use of secukinumab in the treatment of moderate-to-severe psoriasis, including scalp and palmoplantar psoriasis: a 104-week clinical study. Dermatol Ther. 2019;32(5):e13006. https://doi.org/10.1111/dth.13006.
22. Langley RG, Rich P, Menter A, et al. Improvement of scalp and nail lesions with ixekizumab in a phase 2 trial in patients with chronic plaque psoriasis. J Eur Acad Dermatol Venereol. 2015;29(9):1763–70. https://doi.org/10.1111/jdv.12996.
23. Reich K, Leonardi C, Lebwohl M, et al. Sustained response with ixekizumab treatment of moderate-to-severe psoriasis with scalp involvement: results from three phase 3 trials (UNCOVER-1, UNCOVER-2, UNCOVER-3). J Dermatolog Treat. 2017;28(4):282–7. https://doi.org/10.1080/09546634.2016.1249820.
24. Langley RG, Papp K, Gooderham M, et al. Efficacy and safety of continuous every-2-week dosing of ixekizumab over 52 weeks in patients with moderate-to-severe plaque psoriasis in a randomized phase III trial (IXORA-P). Br J Dermatol. 2018;178(6):1315–23. https://doi.org/10.1111/bjd.16426.
25. Papp KA, Blauvelt A, Bukhalo M, et al. Risankizumab versus Ustekinumab for Moderate-to-Severe Plaque Psoriasis. N Engl J Med. 2017;376(16):1551–60. https://doi.org/10.1056/NEJMoa1607017.
26. Dopytalska K, Sobolewski P, Błaszczak A, Szymańska E, Walecka I. Psoriasis in special localizations. Reumatologia. 2018;56(6):392–8. https://doi.org/10.5114/reum.2018.80718.
27. Strober B, Ryan C, van de Kerkhof P, et al. Recategorization of psoriasis severity: Delphi consensus from the International Psoriasis Council. J Am Acad Dermatol. 2020;82(1):117–22. https://doi.org/10.1016/j.jaad.2019.08.026.
28. Ryan C, Menter A, Guenther L, et al. Efficacy and safety of ixekizumab in a randomized, double-blinded, placebo-controlled phase IIIb study of patients with moderate-to-severe genital psoriasis.

Br J Dermatol. 2018;179(4):844–52. https://doi.org/10.1111/bjd.16736.
29. Ješe R, Perdan-Pirkmajer K, Dolenc-Voljč M, Tomšič M. A case of inverse psoriasis successfully treated with adalimumab. Acta Dermatovenerol Alp Pannonica Adriat. 2014;23(1):21–3.
30. Campos MA, Varela P, Baptista A, Moreira AI. Inverse psoriasis treated with ustekinumab. BMJ Case Rep. 2016;2016 https://doi.org/10.1136/bcr-2016-215019.
31. Leonardi C, Langley RG, Papp K, et al. Adalimumab for treatment of moderate to severe chronic plaque psoriasis of the hands and feet: efficacy and safety results from REACH, a randomized, placebo-controlled, double-blind trial. Arch Dermatol. 2011;147(4):429–36. https://doi.org/10.1001/archdermatol.2010.384.
32. Bissonnette R, Poulin Y, Guenther L, Lynde CW, Bolduc C, Nigen S. Treatment of palmoplantar psoriasis with infliximab: a randomized, double-blind placebo-controlled study. J Eur Acad Dermatol Venereol. 2011;25(12):1402–8. https://doi.org/10.1111/j.1468-3083.2011.03984.x.
33. Blauvelt A, Papp KA, Griffiths CEM, et al. Efficacy and safety of guselkumab, an anti-interleukin-23 monoclonal antibody, compared with adalimumab for the continuous treatment of patients with moderate to severe psoriasis: results from the phase III, double-blinded, placebo- and active comparator-controlled VOYAGE 1 trial. J Am Acad Dermatol. 2017;76(3):405–17. https://doi.org/10.1016/j.jaad.2016.11.041.
34. Menter A, Warren RB, Langley RG, et al. Efficacy of ixekizumab compared to etanercept and placebo in patients with moderate-to-severe plaque psoriasis and non-pustular palmoplantar involvement: results from three phase 3 trials (UNCOVER-1, UNCOVER-2 and UNCOVER-3). J Eur Acad Dermatol Venereol. 2017;31(10):1686–92. https://doi.org/10.1111/jdv.14237.
35. Gottlieb A, Sullivan J, van Doorn M, et al. Secukinumab shows significant efficacy in palmoplantar psoriasis: results from GESTURE, a randomized controlled trial. J Am Acad Dermatol. 2017;76(1):70–80. https://doi.org/10.1016/j.jaad.2016.07.058.
36. Paul C, Reich K, Gottlieb AB, et al. Secukinumab improves hand, foot and nail lesions in moderate-to-severe plaque psoriasis: subanalysis of a randomized, double-blind, placebo-controlled, regimen-finding phase 2 trial. J Eur Acad Dermatol Venereol. 2014;28(12):1670–5. https://doi.org/10.1111/jdv.12359.

Comparing Biologic Agents in Treatment of Psoriasis

9

Marwa Hakimi, Megan Mosca, Edward Hadeler, Julie Hong, and Wilson Liao

Introduction

Psoriasis is a chronic, immune-mediated inflammatory skin disease associated with psoriatic arthritis and other comorbidities such as hypertension, diabetes mellitus, hypercholesterolemia, obesity, and metabolic syndrome. Psoriasis occurs in about 3% of the worldwide population and in approximately 7.5 million people in the United States [1]. Currently, without a cure for psoriasis, long-term treatment strategies are imperative. Biologic agents, protein-based therapies that target the immune system, are important treatment options for moderate-to-severe plaque-type psoriasis. Understanding the molecular pathophysiology of psoriasis allows for a targeted approach to therapy. Tumor necrosis factor α (TNF-α) plays a central role in the underlying inflammation of psoriasis, while interleukin (IL)-12 and IL-23 are also key cytokine mediators of psoriasis that induce CD4+ lymphocytes to differentiate into type 1 helper T cells and type 17 helper T cells (the latter of which produce IL-17). Currently, there are eleven FDA-approved biologic options available for psoriasis that target pro-inflammatory cytokines TNF-α, IL-17, IL-12/23, and IL-23. TNF-α inhibitors approved for psoriasis include etanercept, adalimumab, certolizumab pegol, and infliximab. IL-17 inhibitors approved for psoriasis include secukinumab, ixekizumab, and brodalumab. Ustekinumab inhibits both IL-12 and IL-23. Inhibitors of the IL-23 pathway include guselkumab, risankizumab, and tildrakizumab. Biologic agents are chosen on the basis of efficacy, safety, relevant comorbidities, cost, convenience, and patient preference. This chapter examines the efficacy and safety profiles of available psoriasis biologics relative to each other.

Relative Efficacy of Psoriasis Biologics in Head-to-Head Trials

The relative efficacy of psoriasis biologics in head-to-head randomized clinical trials is presented in Table 9.1. Response to therapy is presented as a percentage of patients achieving 75/90/100% improvement in the Psoriasis Area and Severity Index (PASI), percentage of patients

M. Hakimi (✉) · W. Liao
University of California, San Francisco, Department of Dermatology, Psoriasis and Skin Treatment Center, San Francisco, CA, USA
e-mail: marwa.hakimi@ucsf.edu

M. Mosca
University of Nevada, Reno School of Medicine, Reno, NV, USA

E. Hadeler
University of Miami Leonard M. Miller School of Medicine, Miami, FL, USA

J. Hong
Pennsylvania State University College of Medicine, Hershey, PA, USA

N. Brownstone et al. (eds.), *Biologic Therapy for Psoriasis*, Updates in Clinical Dermatology,
https://doi.org/10.1007/978-3-030-92938-1_9

Table 9.1 Head-to-head trials of psoriasis biologic agents

Study Name & Reference	Agent	Comparison drug	N	Time Point	PASI 100	PASI 90	PASI 75	PGA 0/1	DLQI 0/1	Any AE	Most common AE	Discontinuation because of AE
PIECE de Vries AC et al. [2]	Infliximab (INF) 5 mg/kg IV at week 0, 2, 6, 14 and 22	Etanercept (ETA) 50 mg SC twice weekly (biw)	50	Week 12	INF 4% vs ETA 0%	INF 20% vs ETA 0%	INF 76% vs ETA 22%	INF 68% vs ETA 9%	–	–	–	–
				Week 24	INF 8% vs ETA 0%	INF 40% vs ETA 4%	INF 72% vs ETA 35%	INF 76% vs ETA 30%	–	INF 96% vs ETA 100%	INF: common cold/flu vs ETA: skin disease	INF 12% vs ETA 9%
CIMPACT Lebwohl et al. [3]	Certolizumab pegol (CER) 400 mg or 200 mg SC biw (after 400-mg loading doses at weeks 0, 2, and 4) for 16 weeks	Etanercept 50 mg SC biw for 12 weeks	502	Week12	–	–	CER 67% (400 mg) or 61% (200 mg) vs ETA 53%	–	–	CER 49% (400 mg) or 47% (200 mg) vs ETA 46%	CER: nasopharyngitis vs ETA: nasopharyngitis and upper respiratory tract infection (URI)	CER 1% (400 mg) or 1% (200 mg) vs ETA2%
ACCEPT Griffiths et al. [4]	Ustekinumab (UST) 45 mg or 90 mg SC at weeks 0 and 4	Etanercept 50 mg SC biw for 12 weeks	903	Week 12	UST 16% (45 mg) or 26% (90 mg) vs ETA 9%	UST 36% (45 mg) or 45% (90 mg) vs ETA 23%	UST 68% (45 mg) or 74% (90 mg) vs ETA 57%	UST 65% (45 mg) or 71% (90 mg) vs ETA 49%	–	UST 66% (45 mg) or 69% (90 mg) vs ETA 70%	UST: headache vs ETA: injection site reaction	UST 2% (45 mg) or 1% (90 mg) vs ETA 1%
FIXTURE Langley et al. [5]	Secukinumab (SEC) 300 mg or 150 mg SC weekly (qw) for 5 weeks, and then every 4 weeks	Etanercept 50 mg SC biw for 12 weeks, and then qw thereafter	980	Week 12	SEC 24% (300 mg) or 14% (150 mg) vs ETA 4%	SEC 54% (300 mg) or 42% (150 mg) vs ETA 21%	SEC 77% (300 mg) or 67% (150 mg) vs ETA 44%	SEC 63% (300 mg) or 51% (150 mg) vs ETA 27%	SEC 57% (300 mg) or 51% (150 mg) vs ETA 35%	SEC 56% (300 mg) or 58% (150 mg) vs ETA 58%	Nasopharyngitis	SEC 1% (300 mg) or 1% (150 mg) vs ETA 2%

UNCOVER-2 Griffiths et al. [6]	Ixekizumab (IXE) 160 mg SC loading dose and then 80 mg every 4 weeks (4 W), or every 2 weeks (2 W)	Etanercept 50 mg SC biw	1224	Week 12	IXE 31% (4 W) or 41% (2 W) vs ETA 5%	IXE 60% (4 W) or 71% (2 W) vs ETA 19%	IXE 78% (4 W) or 90% (2 W) vs ETA 42%	IXE 73% (4 W) or 83% (2 W) vs ETA 36%	IXE 60% (4 W) or 64% (2 W) vs ETA 34%	IXE 58% (4 W) or 58% (2 W) vs ETA 54%[a]	Injection site reaction[a]	IXE 3% (2 W) vs ETA 7%[a]
UNCOVER-3 Griffiths et al. [6]	Ixekizumab (IXE) 160 mg SC loading dose and then 80 mg every 4 weeks, or every 2 weeks	Etanercept 50 mg SC biw	1346	Week 12	IXE 35% (4 W) or 38% (2 W) vs ETA 7%	IXE 65% (4 W) or 68% (2 W) vs ETA 26%	IXE 84% (4 W) or 87% (2 W) vs ETA 53%	IXE 75% (4 W) or 81% (2 W) vs ETA 42%	IXE 64% (4 W) or 65% (2 W) vs ETA 44%	IXE 58% (4 W) or 58% (2 W) vs ETA 54%[a]	Injection site reaction[a]	IXE 7% (4 W) vs ETA 3%[a]
reSURFACE 2 Reich et al. [7]	Tildrakizumab (TIL) 200 mg or 100 mg SC at weeks 0, 4, and then every 12 weeks	Etanercept 50 mg SC biw for 12 weeks and then qw thereafter	934	Week 12	TIL 12% (200 mg) or 12% (100 mg) vs ETA 5%	TIL 37% (200 mg) or 39% (100 mg) vs ETA 21%	TIL 66% (200 mg) or 61% (100 mg) vs ETA 48%	TIL 59% (200 mg) or 55% (100 mg) vs ETA 48%	TIL 47% (200 mg) or 40% (100 mg) vs ETA 36%	TIL 49% (200 mg) or 44% (100 mg) vs ETA 54%	Nasopharyngitis	TIL 1% (200 mg) or 1% (100 mg) vs ETA 2%
VOYAGE 1 Blauvelt et al. [8].	Guselkumab (GUS) 100 mg SC weeks 0 and 4, and then every 8 weeks	Adalimumab (ADA) 80 mg SC week 0, 40 mg week 1, and then biw	663	Week 16	GUS 37% vs ADA 17%	GUS 73% vs ADA 50%	GUS 91% vs ADA 73%	GUS 85% vs ADA 66%	GUS 56% vs ADA 39%	GUS 52% vs ADA 51%	Nasopharyngitis	GUS 1% vs ADA 1%

(continued)

Table 9.1 (continued)

Study Name & Reference	Agent	Comparison drug	N	Time Point	PASI 100	PASI 90	PASI 75	PGA 0/1	DLQI 0/1	Any AE	Most common AE	Discontinuation because of AE
VOYAGE 2 Reich et al. [9]	Guselkumab (GUS) 100 mg SC weeks 0 and 4, and then every 8 weeks	Adalimumab 80 mg SC week 0, 40 mg week 1, and then biw	744	Week 16	GUS 34% vs ADA 21%	GUS 70% vs ADA 47%	GUS 86% vs ADA 69%	GUS 84% vs ADA 68%	GUS 52% vs ADA 39%	GUS 48% vs ADA 48%	Nasopharyngitis	GUS 1% vs ADA 2%
IMMvent Reich et al. [10]	Risankizumab (RIS) 150 mg SC weeks 0 and 4	Adalimumab 80 mg SC week 0 and then 40 mg biw	605	Week 16	RIS 40% vs ADA 23%	RIS72% vs ADA 47%	RIS 91% vs ADA 72%	RIS 84% vs ADA 60%	RIS 66% vs ADA 49%	RIS 56% vs ADA 57%	Viral URI	RIS 1% vs ADA 2%
CLEAR Thaci et al. [11]	Secukinumab 300 mg SC	Ustekinumab 45 mg SC if ≤100 kg or 90 mg if >100 kg	675	Week 12	SEC 39% vs UST 26%	SEC 73% vs UST 53%	SEC 91% vs UST 79%	SEC 81% vs UST 65%	SEC 66% vs UST 57%	–	–	–
				Week 16	SEC 44% vs UST 28%	SEC 79% vs UST 58%	SEC 93% vs UST 83%	SEC 83% vs UST 68%	SEC 72% vs UST 57%	SEC 64% vs UST 58%	SEC: headache vs UST: nasopharyngitis	SEC 1% vs UST 1%
AMAGINE-2 Lebwohl et al. [12]	Brodalumab (BRO) 210 mg SC or 140 mg biw	Ustekinumab 45 mg SC if ≤100 kg or 90 mg if >100 kg	1522	Week 12	BRO 44% (210 mg) or 26% (140 mg) vs UST 22%	–	BRO 86% (210 mg) or 67% (140 mg) vs UST 70%	BRO 79% (210 mg) or 58% (140 mg) vs UST 61%	–	BRO 58%% (210 mg) or 60% (140 mg) vs UST 59%	BRO: nasopharyngitis vs UST: URI	BRO 1% (210 mg) or 1% (140 mg) vs UST 1%
AMAGINE-3 Lebwohl et al. [12]	Brodalumab (BRO) 210 mg SC or 140 mg biw for 12 weeks[b]	Ustekinumab 45 mg SC if ≤100 kg or 90 mg if >100 kg	1566	Week 12	BRO 37% (210 mg) or 27% (140 mg) vs UST 19%	–	BRO 85% (210 mg) or 69% (140 mg) vs UST 69%	BRO 80% (210 mg) or 60% (140 mg) vs UST 57%	–	BRO 57% (210 mg) or 53% (140 mg) vs UST 54%	BRO: arthralgia (210 mg) or nasopharyngitis (140 mg) vs UST: URI	BRO 1% (210 mg) or 1% (140 mg) vs UST 1%

IXORA-S Reich et al. [13]	Ixekizumab 160 mg SC loading dose and then 80 mg every 2 weeks (2 W) through week 12 and then every 4 weeks thereafter	Ustekinumab 45 mg SC if ≤100 kg or 90 mg if >100 kg	302	Week 12	IXE 36% vs UST 15%	IXE 73% vs UST 42%	IXE 88% vs UST 69%	IXE 84% vs UST 57%	IXE 61% vs UST 45%	–	–	–
				Week 24	IXE 49% vs UST 24%	IXE 83% vs UST 59%	IXE 91% vs UST 82%	IXE 87% vs UST 69%	IXE 66% vs UST 53%	IXE 70% vs UST 75%	Nasopharyngitis	IXE 2% vs UST 1%
NCT02054481 Papp et al. [14]	Risankizumab single 18 mg SC dose week 0 or 90 mg or 180 mg at weeks 0, 4, and 16	Ustekinumab 45 mg SC if ≤100 kg or 90 mg if >100 kg	166	Week 12	RIS 14% (18 mg) or 41% (90 mg) or 48% (180 mg) vs UST 18%	RIS 33% (18 mg) or 73% (90 mg) or 81% (180 mg) vs UST 40%	RIS 63% (18 mg) or 98% (90 mg) or 88% (180 mg) vs UST 72%	RIS 58% (18 mg) or 90% (90 mg) or 88% (180 mg) vs UST 62%	RIS 42% (18 mg) or 71% (90 mg) or 73% (180 mg) vs UST 53%	RIS 81% (18 mg) or 80% (90 mg) or 69% (180 mg) vs UST 72%[c]	Nasopharyngitis[c]	RIS 2% (18 mg) or 2% (90 mg) or 0% (180 mg) vs UST 2%[c]
IXORA-R Blauvelt et al. [15]	Ixekizumab 160 mg SC loading dose and then 80 mg every 2 weeks	Guselkumab 100 mg SC at weeks 0, 4, and 12	1027	Week 12	IXE 41% vs GUS 25%	–	–	IXE 42% vs GUS 25%[d]	–	IXE 56% vs GUS 55%[e]	IXE: Injection site reaction vs GUS: URI[e]	IXE 2% vs GUS 2%[e]
ECLIPSE Reich et al. [16]	Guselkumab 100 mg SC at weeks 0 and 4 and then every 8 weeks	Secukinumab 300 mg SC at weeks 0, 1, 2, 3, and 4, and then every 4 weeks	1048	Week12	–	GUS 69% vs SEC 76%	GUS 89% vs SEC 92%	–	–	–	–	–
				Week 48	GUS 58% vs SEC 48%	GUS 84% vs SEC 70%	–	GUS 85% vs SEC 75%	–	GUS 78% vs SEC 82%	Nasopharyngitis	GUS 2% vs SEC 2%

[a]Adverse event data for [a]UNCOVER-2 and UNCOVER-3 were pooled by original authors
[b]After 12 weeks randomized to 4 groups: 210 mg biw, 140 biw, 140 mg monthly, or 140 mg every 8 weeks for weeks 12–52
[c]Reported as through week 48
[d]PGA score of 0 only reported
[e]Reported as through week 24

achieving a Physician Global Assessment (PGA) of 0 or 1 (clear or almost clear skin), and the percentage of patients achieving a Dermatology Life Quality Index (DLQI) score of 0 or 1 (no impact of skin disease on quality of life).

Etanercept as the Reference Biologic

Biologic agents that inhibit TNF-α (infliximab and certolizumab pegol), IL-12/23 (ustekinumab), IL-17 (secukinumab and ixekizumab), and IL-23 (tildrakizumab) have been compared to TNF-α inhibitor, etanercept, which was FDA-approved for use in psoriasis in 2004 [2–5]. Etanercept is typically dosed 50 mg subcutaneously twice weekly for the first 12 weeks and then 50 mg subcutaneously weekly. The newer biologic agents all have less frequent dosing than etanercept. All of these biologic agents were more effective in achieving PASI 75 than etanercept at week 12.

Infliximab showed greater efficacy and more rapid onset of action than etanercept at weeks 12 and 24 based on percentage of patients reaching PASI 75/90/100. Furthermore, all patients taking infliximab reached PASI 50 by week 24. A majority (76%) of patients receiving infliximab achieved clear or almost clear skin based on physician assessment at week 24 in contrast to only 30% of patients receiving etanercept [2]. Additionally, a longer mean duration of remission was observed in the infliximab group compared to the etanercept group, 15.5 weeks versus 13.7 weeks, after study medication discontinuation at week 24. Although infliximab and etanercept both inhibit TNF-α, they employ different strategies to neutralize TNF-α, which may explain the many differences between these agents.

Similarly, the efficacy of certolizumab pegol, a TNF-α inhibitor approved for use by the FDA in 2008, was shown to be superior to etanercept in achieving PASI 75 at week 12 [3].

The efficacy of ustekinumab with two injections at a dose of 45 or 90 mg was superior to that of high-dose etanercept with twice-weekly injections during a 12-week period. Moreover, 48.9% of patients who did not have a response to etanercept had at least 75% improvement in PASI at week 12 after crossover to ustekinumab [4]. The median time to recurrence after discontinuing treatment at week 12 if subjects achieved a PGA score of 0–2 was longer for ustekinumab, 14.4 weeks and 18.1 weeks among those who received 45 mg and 90 mg respectively, compared to 7.3 weeks for those who received etanercept. Importantly, among those who discontinued treatment with ustekinumab, 84.4% achieved a PGA score of 0–2 within 12 weeks after retreatment. Biologic discontinuation is a reality that both providers and patients are faced with. Biologic resistance over time is also a relevant consideration when choosing among the different agents. Antibodies to ustekinumab were developed in 3.8% of patients with the majority having low titers.

The IL-17 inhibitor secukinumab, at doses of either 300 mg or 150 mg, was superior to etanercept in efficacy based on the rates of response according to PASI 75/90/100 through week 52. A significantly higher proportion of patients receiving secukinumab in each dose group achieved clear or almost clear skin by week 12 [5]. These findings were supported by a higher proportion of patients in the secukinumab group achieving a Dermatology Life Quality Index score of 0 or 1.

Similarly, ixekizumab, an IL-17 inhibitor FDA-approved in 2017, given at either 80 mg every 2 weeks or every 4 weeks after a 160 mg loading dose, was superior in efficacy as measured by PASI 75/90/100 than etanercept at week 12 in two independent studies [6]. A majority of patients on both regimens of ixekizumab achieved PASI 90 by week 12, which is in contrast to the majority of patients in the etanercept group only achieving PASI 75 during the same time frame. Furthermore, a majority of patients receiving ixekizumab at either dosing regimens indicated that their psoriasis had no impact on their quality of life by week 12. As expected, more patients that received the more frequent dosing of ixekizumab at every 2 weeks versus every 4 weeks achieved complete clearance, PASI 100, by week 12.

Lastly, the IL-23 inhibitor tildrakizumab was shown to be superior to etanercept in the treatment of moderate-to-severe chronic plaque psoriasis. A greater proportion of patients receiving tildrakizumab reported no effect of psoriasis on quality of life by week 12 than etanercept patients. Both tildrakizumab regimens, 200 mg and 100 mg, improved psoriasis with a majority achieving PASI 90 by week 28 [7].

Adalimumab as the Reference Biologic

Newer biologics agents that inhibit IL-23 (guselkumab and risankizumab) have been compared to the TNF-α inhibitor, adalimumab, which was FDA-approved for use in psoriasis in 2002 [8–10]. Adalimumab is typically dosed at 80 mg subcutaneously at week 0, 40 mg at week 1, and then 40 mg subcutaneously biweekly. Both guselkumab and risankizumab were more effective in achieving PASI 75 than adalimumab at week 12.

Guselkumab was superior to adalimumab in efficacy with significantly higher proportions achieving PASI 90 and PASI 75 at week 16 and improvement in patient-reported outcomes through week 48 [8]. Additionally, by week 24 more than half (52%) of patients in the guselkumab group were completely clear compared to only 29% in the adalimumab group in the same time frame. VOYAGE 2 confirmed that guselkumab was superior to adalimumab in efficacy even with interrupted treatment [9]. The study design included a randomized withdrawal and retreatment period during weeks 28–72; this is important to analyze as treatment gaps often occur in clinical practice. For the withdrawal group, the median time to lose PASI 90 was 23 weeks after the last dose of guselkumab.

Similarly, risankizumab was superior to adalimumab in efficacy with significantly higher proportions achieving PASI 90 starting at week 8, and by week 16, it was 72% of patients compared to 47% in the adalimumab group [10]. Although more than half of the adalimumab group achieved a PGA of clear or almost clear by week 16, less than half of the adalimumab group reported that psoriasis had no effect on their life. Switching from adalimumab to risankizumab was superior to continuing adalimumab after week 16 in achieving PASI 90 by week 44 in patients with an intermediate response to adalimumab (PASI ≥50 to <90).

Ustekinumab as the Reference Biologic

Blockade of key mediators of psoriasis, IL-12 and IL-23, by ustekinumab has been compared to biologics agents that inhibit IL-17 (ixekizumab, brodalumab, and secukinumab) and IL-23 (risankizumab). Both the anti-IL-17 and anti-IL-23 biologic agents were more effective in achieving PASI 75 than ustekinumab.

A significantly higher proportion of patients achieved PASI 90 at week 16 in the secukinumab group (79%) than those in ustekinumab group (58%) [11]. Consistent with its clinical efficacy, more patients in the secukinumab group reported that psoriasis had no effect on their lives (72% vs 57%) at week 16. Clinical responses were not only greater in the secukinumab group, but also occurred earlier throughout the 16-week treatment period.

The 210 mg dose of brodalumab was superior to ustekinumab in efficacy with higher proportions achieving PASI 100 and PASI 75 at week 12 in both AMAGINE-2 and 3. Although the 140 mg dose of brodalumab was superior to ustekinumab in achieving PASI 100 at week 12, slightly more patients in the ustekinumab group achieved PGA 0/1 (61% vs 58%) and PASI 75 (70% vs 67%) in AMAGINE-2, while equal proportions of patients achieved PASI 75 (69%) in AMAGINE-3 [12]. In both studies, the median time to PASI 75 response was shorter with either brodalumab dose (4 weeks in the 210 mg group and 6 weeks in the 140 mg group) than with ustekinumab (8 weeks).

Ixekizumab was superior to ustekinumab in efficacy with higher proportions achieving PASI 100/90/75 and PGA 0/1 at weeks 12 and 24, which was consistent with more patients reporting that psoriasis had no effect on their lives in the ixekizumab group compared to ustekinumab. At week 12, 74% of patients receiving ixekizumab achieved PASI 90 compared to 42% of patients receiving ustekinumab. Furthermore, ixekizumab had faster onset of action with patients achieving PASI 100 by week 4 compared with ustekinumab (6.6% vs 0% $P < 0.001$) [13]. Of note, ustekinumab efficacy was slightly lower in this study than data reported in the CLEAR study, which was possibly related to the differences in patient populations [11].

Similarly, risankizumab at both doses (90 mg and 180 mg) was superior to ustekinumab in efficacy with significantly higher proportions achieving PASI 90 at week 12. PASI 100 was achieved in 41% of patients in the 90 mg risankizumab group and 48% of patients in the 180 mg risankizumab group, compared with 18% of patients who received ustekinumab at week 12. Higher dose of risankizumab was superior to lower dose in all response measures, except for PASI 75, with 98% of patients in the 90 mg group achieving PASI 75 compared to 88% in the 180 mg group [14]. Ustekinumab was superior in all outcome measures at week 12 than a single dose of risankizumab 180 mg. Notably, more than half of patients that received the single dose of 180 mg risankizumab achieved PASI 75 and PGA score of 0 or 1 at week 12.

Guselkumab as the Reference Biologic

Blockade of IL-23 by guselkumab has been compared to ixekizumab, an IL-17 inhibitor. Ixekizumab was superior to guselkumab in efficacy at clearing skin as measured by PASI 100 (41% vs 25% $P < 0.001$) and PGA 0 (24% vs 25%) at week 12 [15]. More patients who achieved PASI 75 by week 2 in both group groups reported that psoriasis did not have an effect on their quality of life at week 2 compared with those who did not achieve PASI 75 at this time point, thus indicating a significance in achieving early improvements in PASI.

Secukinumab as the Reference Biologic

Blockade of IL-23 by guselkumab has been compared to IL-17 inhibitor, secukinumab. Although secukinumab was superior in achieving PASI 90/75 at week 12, guselkumab was superior in efficacy as measured by the proportion of patients achieving PASI 100/90 and PGA 0/1 than secukinumab at week 48 [16]. Thus, guselkumab showed superiority in long-term efficacy.

Relative Efficacy of Psoriasis Biologics Based on Network Meta-Analyses (NMA)

NMA Efficacy at 8–24 Weeks

Biologic agents were ranked based on efficacy using surface under the cumulative ranking (SUCRA) curve method in many of the network meta-analyses [17–20]. Although the NMAs had differing results, risankizumab, ixekizumab, and brodalumab were generally among the top three most efficacious agents reported in these studies (Table 9.2). On the other end of the spectrum, TNF-alpha inhibitors and ustekinumab generally had lower efficacy than the other biologic agents, with the exception of infliximab. These results are consistent with the data reported from head-to-head trials presented above. Interestingly, in one study, ranking for PASI 90 using SUCRA suggested that infliximab was the most efficacious treatment, followed by ixekizumab, risankizumab, guselkumab, secukinumab, brodalumab, adalimumab, tildrakizumab, ustekinumab, certolizumab pegol, and then etanercept [17]. However, in another NMA, infliximab was not ranked as best, with the anti-IL-23 and anti-IL-17 agents, risankizumab and ixekizumab, performing better [18]. PASI response rates in the induction phase were shown to be highest for risankizumab and ixekizumab in other analyses as well [19]. Both are the most recent FDA-approved agent within their class. Risankizumab was also shown to have the highest PASI response rate in the long term [19]. Further analysis found risankizumab to be significantly superior at achieving all PASI response levels compared to other therapies with the exception of guselkumab and brodalumab [20].

Table 9.2 Network meta-analyses of psoriasis biologic agents

Reference	Efficacy ranking	Safety ranking
Sbidian et al. [17]	PASI 90 induction phase (8–24 weeks) performed with SUCRA: INF > IXE > RIS > GUS > SEC > BRO>ADA > TIL > UST > CER > ETA	Serious adverse events (SAEs) performed with SUCRA: RIS > CER > TIL > UST > ETA>GUS > ADA > BRO>INF > IXE > SEC
Tada et al. [18]	PASI 90 induction phase (10–16 weeks) performed with SUCRA: RIS > BRO>IXE > GUS > SEC > INF > ADA > UST	–
Armstrong et al. [19]	PASI 90 induction phase (10–16 weeks) performed with SUCRA: IXE > RIS > BRO>GUS > SEC > INF > CER > UST > ADA > TIL > ETA	–
Yasmeen et al. [20]	PASI 90 induction phase (10–16 weeks) performed with SUCRA: RIS > BRO>GUS > IXE > SEC > UST > INF>CER[a]>ADA > CER[b] > ETA	–
Shear et al. [21]	–	SAEs (12–16 weeks) performed with SUCRA: CER[b] > RIS > ETA>BRO>ADA > TIL[d] > UST > INF > GUS>CER[a]>IXE > SEC>TIL[c] AEs leading to treatment discontinuation performed with SUCRA: RIS > TIL[d] > GUS > UST > ETA>ADA > SEC > BRO>TIL[c]>IXE>CER[a]>INF > CER[b]

Note: SUCRA is expressed as a percentage between 0 (treatment is the worst) and 100% (treatment is the best)

[a]Certolizumab at 400 mg q2week vs [b]certolizumab without a notation is dosing for weight < 90 kg at 400 mg at weeks 0, 2, and 4, and then 200 mg every 2 week

[c]Tildrakizumab at 200 mg at weeks 0 and 4, then Q12 weeks vs [d]tildrakizumab standard dosing at 100 mg at week 0 and 4, and then 100 mg every 12 weeks

Relative Safety of Psoriasis Biologics in Head-to-Head Trials

Although it is useful to understand the relative efficacies of biologic treatments for psoriasis, consideration of drug side effects also plays an important role in treatment selection. Overall, biologic agents were well tolerated in the treatment of patients with moderate-to-severe chronic plaque psoriasis for the timeline of the trials as shown in Table 9.1.

Etanercept as the Reference Biologic

Although patients receiving etanercept experienced some adverse events, significantly more adverse events occurred in the infliximab group (201 vs 148, $P = 0.03$) [2]. In both groups, most adverse events were noted to be mild with common cold/flu and skin disease being the most common adverse event. The actual treatment-related adverse events (probably or definitely) were much lower, 16% in the infliximab group and 12% in the etanercept group. Notably, increased infusion reactions and antibody formation occurred when restarting infliximab after a treatment-free interval of more than 16 weeks.

While fewer patients receiving certolizumab pegol discontinued treatment due to adverse events compared to those receiving etanercept, both groups had comparable safety through week 12 [3].

For the IL-12/23 inhibitor ustekinumab, safety rates and types of adverse events were similar to anti-TNF-α agent, etanercept in short-term treatment. Furthermore, both agents were comparable in the proportion of patients that experienced infections and the proportion that discontinued treatment because of adverse events. A notable exception was more injection site reactions with etanercept, which may be partly explained by the increased number of injections received among that group [4].

One quarter of patients in the etanercept group experienced infections by week 12 of induction, compared with 27% and 31% of patients receiving secukinumab at 300 mg and 150 mg, respectively. During the entire treatment period, candida infections were more common in secukinumab, but it did not result in discontinuation of the study drug. More patients in the etanercept group discontinued medication due to adverse events compared with secukinumab [5].

Most adverse events were mild or moderate in severity for both the IL-17 inhibitor, ixekizumab, and etanercept groups with injection site reactions being the most common. Patients receiving ixekizumab every 2 weeks had similar rates of injection site reactions to those receiving etanercept, 17% and 16%, respectively, while those receiving ixekizumab every 4 weeks had the least at 13% [6]. Furthermore, rates of serious adverse events were comparable across study groups, 2% or fewer patients in each treatment group. However, ixekizumab and etanercept treatment groups were noted to have different discontinuation rates, 3% of patients receiving ixekizumab every 2 weeks discontinued treatment compared with 7% of patients receiving etanercept (UNCOVER-2), while 7% of patients receiving ixekizumab at every 4 weeks discontinued treatment [5]. There were no significant differences in the specific reason for discontinuation between the treatment groups.

In both the tildrakizumab and etanercept groups, nasopharyngitis was the most common adverse event. The proportion of patients in the different treatment groups with serious adverse events was low. Additionally, a similar and low proportion of patients discontinued treatment because of adverse event [7].

Adalimumab as the Reference Biologic

Types of adverse events and serious adverse events were comparable between the guselkumab and adalimumab groups through week 48. However, more patients experienced injection site reactions in the adalimumab group, likely related to the increased number of injections compared to guselkumab [8, 9]. Both guselkumab studies showed that selectively targeting IL-23, a key regulator of Th17 cell survival and differentiation, results in a higher degree of efficacy while also maintaining a favorable safety profile compared with TNF-α blockade.

Both risankizumab and adalimumab groups had low and comparable frequencies of treatment-emergent adverse events and adverse events leading to drug discontinuation at week 16. Viral upper respiratory tract infection and headache were among the most frequently reported adverse events in both groups. Among adalimumab intermediate responders, more patients reported adverse events when switched to risankizumab (75%) compared to those that remained on adalimumab (66%) from week 16–44 [10].

Ustekinumab as the Reference Biologic

Secukinumab and ustekinumab exhibited a similar safety profile through week 16 with 3% experiencing nonfatal serious adverse events and 1% of each group discontinuing medication because of adverse events [11]. Headache and nasopharyngitis were the most frequently reported adverse events in both groups. IL-17 plays a role in host defense involving mucocutaneous microbial surveillance, thus why more candida infections are observed. Although twelve cases of mild-to-moderate localized mucosal or cutaneous candida infections were reported, none led to treatment discontinuation.

The most frequently reported adverse events in both brodalumab and ustekinumab groups were nasopharyngitis, upper respiratory tract infection, headache, and arthralgia. Rates and types of serious adverse events were comparable across study groups, 2% or fewer patients in each treatment group in both studies [12]. As expected, more candida infections occurred with brodalumab and then with ustekinumab through week 12.

Through 24 weeks, nasopharyngitis was the most common treatment-emergent adverse effect in both ustekinumab and ixekizumab treatment groups. During this time, 4% of ixekizumab group experienced severe treatment-emergent adverse events compared to 6% in the ustekinumab group [13]. Less than 2% of patients in each group discontinued treatment because of an adverse event.

During the 48-week treatment period, adverse events occurred in a larger proportion of patients receiving lower dose risankizumab (80% in 90 mg group), compared to higher dose risankizumab (69% in 180 mg group) and ustekinumab (72%) [14]. Nasopharyngitis was the most common adverse event occurring in all treatment groups. One patient discontinued treatment because of an adverse event in the 90 mg risankizumab group and ustekinumab group. However, no patients in the higher dose risankizumab (180 mg) group discontinued treatment.

Guselkumab as the Reference Biologic

Both guselkumab and ixekizumab groups reported the same low frequencies of serious adverse events (3% in both) and discontinuation because of adverse events (2% in both) through week 24 [15]. Although injection site reactions were the most common adverse event in the ixekizumab group, these reactions were all mild to moderate in severity.

Secukinumab as the Reference Biologic

Overall, more adverse events were reported in the secukinumab group, 82% compared to 78% in guselkumab group through week 48 [16]. Nasopharyngitis was the most common adverse event reported in both the guselkumab and secukinumab groups. As expected, more candida infections occurred in the secukinumab group. Serious adverse events occurred in 7% of patients receiving secukinumab and 6% of patients receiving guselkumab. In each group, 2% of patients discontinued treatment because of an adverse event.

Relative Safety of Psoriasis Biologics in Network Meta-Analyses (NMA)

Biologic agents were ranked based on adverse events using surface under the cumulative ranking (SUCRA) curve method in many of the network meta-analyses [17, 21]. Analysis of serious adverse events with SUCRA indicates that IL-23 inhibitors as a class were associated with the best safety profile, followed by IL-12/23 inhibitors, TNF-α inhibitors, and then IL-17 inhibitors (Table 9.2). Ranking analysis at a drug level for serious adverse events using SUCRA indicated that risankizumab was associated with the best safety profile, followed by certolizumab, tildrakizumab, ustekinumab, etanercept, guselkumab, adalimumab, brodalumab, infliximab, and ixekizumab, followed by secukinumab [17]. Another NMA also indicated that the risankizumab was associated with low rates of safety events in the short term along with the other agents in the anti-IL-23 class (guselkumab and tildrakizumab) [21]. Furthermore, risankizumab was associated with a lower probability of treatment discontinuation because of adverse events. Long-term data suggest that risankizumab has the lowest rate of any adverse events, serious adverse events, and adverse events leading to discontinuations. Taking this together with the NMA efficacy rankings based on PASI 90, risankizumab appears to both be highly efficacious and safe.

Conclusion

Moderate-to-severe plaque psoriasis requires treatment with phototherapy or systemic therapies such as biologic immune modifying agents. Although currently there is no cure of psoriasis, the availability of biologic agents has reduced some of the challenges of managing patients with extensive or recalcitrant disease. To facilitate the selection of appropriate biologic agent, it is important to assess multiple aspects of each agent, including efficacy and safety. There is ample evidence of not only short-term and long-term efficacy, but also tolerability of biologic medications. The data presented here can help practitioners select biologic agents based on relative efficacy and safety rating.

Take-Home Points

- In direct comparison, IL-17 and IL-23 inhibitors are generally more effective than IL-12/23 and TNF-(inhibitors
  - Brodalumab, ixekizumab, secukinumab (IL17 inhibitors), and risankizumab (IL-23 inhibitor) were more effective than ustekinumab (IL-12/23 inhibitor)
  - Risankizumab and guselkumab (IL-23 inhibitor) were more effective than adalimumab (TNF-(inhibitor)
  - Secukinumab, ixekizumab (IL-17 inhibitors), tildrakizumab (IL-23 inhibitor), ustekinumab (IL-12/23 inhibitor), certolizumab, and infliximab (TNF-(inhibitor) were more effective than etanercept (TNF-(inhibitor)
- In network meta-analyses: risankizumab, ixekizumab, and brodalumab were generally the most effective in achieving PASI 90
- In network meta-analyses: risankizumab, certolizumab, tildrakizumab, ustekinumab, etanercept, and guselkumab had the fewest serious adverse events

References

1. Menter A, Gottlieb A, Feldman SR, Van Voorhees AS, et al. Guidelines of care for the management of psoriasis and psoriatic arthritis: section 1. Overview of psoriasis and guidelines of care for the treatment of psoriasis with biologics. J Am Acad Dermatol. 2008;58(5):826–50.
2. de Vries AC, Thio HB, de Kort WJ, et al. A prospective randomized controlled trial comparing infliximab and etanercept in patients with moderate-to-severe chronic plaque-type psoriasis: the Psoriasis Infliximab vs. Etanercept Comparison Evaluation (PIECE) study. Br J Dermatol. 2017;176(3):624–33. https://doi.org/10.1111/bjd.14867.

3. Lebwohl M, Blauvelt A, Paul C, et al. Certolizumab pegol for the treatment of chronic plaque psoriasis: results through 48 weeks of a phase 3, multicenter, randomized, double-blind, etanercept- and placebo-controlled study (CIMPACT). J Am Acad Dermatol. 2018;79(2):266–276.e5. https://doi.org/10.1016/j.jaad.2018.04.013.
4. Griffiths CE, Strober BE, van de Kerkhof P, et al. Comparison of ustekinumab and etanercept for moderate-to-severe psoriasis. N Engl J Med. 2010;362(2):118–28. https://doi.org/10.1056/NEJMoa0810652.
5. Langley RG, Elewski BE, Lebwohl M, et al. Secukinumab in plaque psoriasis--results of two phase 3 trials. N Engl J Med. 2014;371(4):326–38. https://doi.org/10.1056/NEJMoa1314258.
6. Griffiths CE, Reich K, Lebwohl M, et al. Comparison of ixekizumab with etanercept or placebo in moderate-to-severe psoriasis (UNCOVER-2 and UNCOVER-3): results from two phase 3 randomised trials. Lancet. 2015;386(9993):541–51. https://doi.org/10.1016/S0140-6736(15)60125-8.
7. Reich K, Papp KA, Blauvelt A, et al. Tildrakizumab versus placebo or etanercept for chronic plaque psoriasis (reSURFACE 1 and reSURFACE 2): results from two randomised controlled, phase 3 trials [published correction appears in Lancet. 2017 Jul 15;390(10091):230]. Lancet. 2017;390(10091):276–88. https://doi.org/10.1016/S0140-6736(17)31279-5.
8. Blauvelt A, Papp KA, Griffiths CE, et al. Efficacy and safety of guselkumab, an anti-interleukin-23 monoclonal antibody, compared with adalimumab for the continuous treatment of patients with moderate to severe psoriasis: results from the phase III, double-blinded, placebo- and active comparator-controlled VOYAGE 1 trial. J Am Acad Dermatol. 2017;76(3):405–17. https://doi.org/10.1016/j.jaad.2016.11.041.
9. Reich K, Armstrong AW, Foley P, et al. Efficacy and safety of guselkumab, an anti-interleukin-23 monoclonal antibody, compared with adalimumab for the treatment of patients with moderate to severe psoriasis with randomized withdrawal and retreatment: results from the phase III, double-blind, placebo- and active comparator-controlled VOYAGE 2 trial. J Am Acad Dermatol. 2017;76(3):418–31. https://doi.org/10.1016/j.jaad.2016.11.042.
10. Reich K, Gooderham M, Thaçi D, et al. Risankizumab compared with adalimumab in patients with moderate-to-severe plaque psoriasis (IMMvent): a randomised, double-blind, active-comparator-controlled phase 3 trial [published correction appears in Lancet. 2019 Jul 16]. Lancet. 2019;394(10198):576–86. https://doi.org/10.1016/S0140-6736(19)30952-3.
11. Thaçi D, Blauvelt A, Reich K, et al. Secukinumab is superior to ustekinumab in clearing skin of subjects with moderate to severe plaque psoriasis: CLEAR, a randomized controlled trial. J Am Acad Dermatol. 2015;73(3):400–9. https://doi.org/10.1016/j.jaad.2015.05.013.
12. Lebwohl M, Strober B, Menter A, et al. Phase 3 studies comparing Brodalumab with Ustekinumab in psoriasis. N Engl J Med. 2015;373(14):1318–28. https://doi.org/10.1056/NEJMoa1503824.
13. Reich K, Pinter A, Lacour JP, et al. Comparison of ixekizumab with ustekinumab in moderate-to-severe psoriasis: 24-week results from IXORA-S, a phase III study. Br J Dermatol. 2017;177(4):1014–23. https://doi.org/10.1111/bjd.15666.
14. Papp KA, Blauvelt A, Bukhalo M, et al. Risankizumab versus Ustekinumab for Moderate-to-Severe Plaque Psoriasis. N Engl J Med. 2017;376(16):1551–60. https://doi.org/10.1056/NEJMoa1607017.
15. Blauvelt A, Papp K, Gottlieb A, et al. A head-to-head comparison of ixekizumab vs. guselkumab in patients with moderate-to-severe plaque psoriasis: 12-week efficacy, safety and speed of response from a randomized, double-blinded trial. Br J Dermatol. 2020;182(6):1348–58. https://doi.org/10.1111/bjd.18851.
16. Reich K, Armstrong AW, Langley RG, et al. Guselkumab versus secukinumab for the treatment of moderate-to-severe psoriasis (ECLIPSE): results from a phase 3, randomised controlled trial. Lancet. 2019;394(10201):831–9. https://doi.org/10.1016/S0140-6736(19)31773.
17. Sbidian E, Chaimani A, Afach S, et al. Systemic pharmacological treatments for chronic plaque psoriasis: a network meta-analysis. Cochrane Database Syst Rev. 2020;1(1):CD011535. https://doi.org/10.1002/14651858.CD011535.pub3.
18. Tada Y, Watanabe R, Noma H, Kanai Y, Nomura T, Kaneko K. Short-term effectiveness of biologics in patients with moderate-to-severe plaque psoriasis: a systematic review and network meta-analysis. J Dermatol Sci. 2020;99(1):53–61. https://doi.org/10.1016/j.jdermsci.2020.06.003.
19. Armstrong AW, Soliman AM, Betts KA, et al. Comparative efficacy and relative ranking of biologics and Oral therapies for moderate-to-severe plaque psoriasis: a network meta-analysis. Dermatol Ther (Heidelb). 2021;11(3):885–905. https://doi.org/10.1007/s13555-021-00511-1.
20. Yasmeen N, Sawyer LM, Malottki K, Levin LÅ, Didriksen Apol E, Jemec GB. Targeted therapies for patients with moderate-to-severe psoriasis: a systematic review and network meta-analysis of PASI response at 1 year [published online ahead of print, 2020 Apr 2]. J Dermatolog Treat. 2020:1–15. https://doi.org/10.1080/09546634.2020.1743811.
21. Shear NH, Betts KA, Soliman AM, et al. Comparative safety and benefit-risk profile of biologics and oral treatment for moderate-to-severe plaque psoriasis: a network meta-analysis of clinical trial data. J Am Acad Dermatol. 2021;85(3):572–81. https://doi.org/10.1016/j.jaad.2021.02.057.

10 Long-Term Registry Data for Psoriasis Biologics

Deborah Cull, Joseph Pena, Esther A. Balogh, Caitlin G. Purvis, and Steven R. Feldman

Introduction

Biologics have revolutionized the treatment of psoriasis. In clinical trials for psoriasis, biologics are highly effective and very safe, but clinical trials may not be informative about rare risks, long-term safety and efficacy, or safety in patients who would be ineligible for the trial. Clinical data registries are complementary to clinical trials, addressing some limitations through observational study methods to collect data. Long-term registry data for psoriasis biologics have been used to monitor real-world patient adherence, persistence, drug efficacy, adverse outcomes, and many other parameters. These data can be analyzed to determine which biologic treatments have better real-world efficacy for psoriasis and which psoriasis treatments are associated with a higher rate of adverse events (AEs). In addition to this, registry data can be analyzed to determine patient adherence and persistence to specific drugs. According to recent data from psoriasis registries, biologics are associated with a lower rate of AEs compared to older systemic therapies. Psoriasis registries are informative about real-world efficacy and confirm the excellent safety profile of biologic therapies.

D. Cull (✉) · J. Pena · E. A. Balogh · C. G. Purvis
Center for Dermatology Research, Department of Dermatology, Wake Forest School of Medicine, Winston-Salem, NC, USA
e-mail: dcull@wakehealth.edu; brundage@alumni.princeton.edu

S. R. Feldman
Center for Dermatology Research, Department of Dermatology, Wake Forest School of Medicine, Winston-Salem, NC, USA

Department of Pathology, Wake Forest School of Medicine, Winston-Salem, NC, USA

Department of Social Sciences & Health Policy, Wake Forest School of Medicine, Winston-Salem, NC, USA

Department of Dermatology, University of Southern Denmark, Odense, Denmark

The Importance of Registry Studies

History of Biologic Therapy

In the United States, biologic agents were first approved to treat moderate-to-severe plaque psoriasis by the Food and Drug Administration (FDA) in 2003 (alefacept in January 2003 and efalizumab in October 2003) [1, 2]. Before this approval, alefacept and efalizumab improved plaque and psoriatic arthritis in randomized controlled trials (RCTs). The rate of patients achieving at least a 50% reduction in the Psoriasis Area and Severity Index (PASI) was 22% higher in those taking alefacept ($n = 507$) and 44.6% more in patients taking efalizumab ($n = 369$) compared to those taking the placebo ($p < 0.001$). Soon

N. Brownstone et al. (eds.), *Biologic Therapy for Psoriasis*, Updates in Clinical Dermatology,
https://doi.org/10.1007/978-3-030-92938-1_10

after, in 2004, etanercept was approved for the treatment of psoriasis [1, 2].

Many biologics have been studied, such as tumor necrosis factor-α (TNF-α inhibitors (etanercept, adalimumab, certolizumab, infliximab), interleukin-17 (IL-17) inhibitors (secukinumab, ixekizumab, and brodalumab), IL-12/23 inhibitors (ustekinumab), and IL-23 inhibitors (guselkumab, tildrakizumab, and risankizumab) [3]. These biologic agents have a variety of mechanisms of action, increasing the treatment options beyond what has been historically available prior to their development [4, 5].

Long-Term Risks of Biologics for Psoriasis Treatment

The long-term risks of biologic therapy for the treatment of psoriasis have not been investigated fully through RCTs. AEs are rare; however, events leading to discontinuation of biologics may include injection site reactions, infusion reactions, infection, malignancy, tuberculosis reactivation, lupus-like symptoms, iritis, cardiac, and neurologic AEs [6, 7]. The significance of these AEs has been studied with RCTs, which compare biologic therapy to older systemic therapies and a placebo. The short time frame and close patient follow-up of RCTs make it difficult to predict the outcomes of biologic therapy in a real-life clinical setting. Psoriasis registries such as Psoriasis Longitudinal Assessment Registry (PSOLAR), British Association of Dermatologists Biologic and Immunomodulators Register (BADBIR), and the Psonet initiative were created to specifically address the long-term benefits and risks of these biologic therapies for psoriasis. Their data are more indicative of patients' real-life behavior compared to RCTs with their short timeline, inclusion/exclusion criteria, close consistent follow-up, and participants' heightened perception of being observed [8].

How Biologic Registries Are Conducted

Data registries are organized into subtypes by areas of interest such as specific disease, drug type, drug class, pregnancy exposure, and many more [9]. Registries enroll patients voluntarily and set a predetermined goal for the number of patients necessary to collect data on a disease of interest [1, 10]. These data—which include clinical and nonclinical information such as demographics, medical and family history, and medical treatment details—are collected periodically with medical appointments and/or the receipt of medication from the pharmacy. For example, if a participant is seen by the physician for medication management every 6 months, the data could be collected on a six-month basis [10, 11]. Inclusion criteria are determined by the investigators, and diagnosis of psoriasis is the primary criterion for inclusion when investigating the biologic treatment of psoriasis. Additional criteria include the ability to attend appointments and agreement to take the drug of interest. Exclusion criteria can vary based on the registry study and may exclude participants from certain groups such as patients who have previously participated in certain clinical trials, those who cannot or refuse to consent, or those who are unable to participate for a specific time frame [12].

Some registries have cohorts on biologic therapies and separate cohorts on nonbiologic therapies. These may require patients on nonbiologic therapies to be biologically naive, i.e., having never previously used biologic treatment [11]. Within these studies, the first data points are collected on the first appointment after consent and enrollment into the registry database. Data points of interest may include demographics such as race and gender, medication history, disease history, family history of disease, treatment history for the disease of interest, and progression of the disease of interest [12]. Outcome information is obtained as patients are followed continually as part of the registry and may include serious harm or death, the onset of a new illness, disability, infections, neurologic concerns, pregnancy issues, malignancy, new-onset autoimmune disease, cardiovascular events, vaccine injuries, immunosuppression, hepatotoxicity, and changes in psychiatric diagnosis. This is not a comprehensive list, and registries vary in data collected and methods of collection [11, 12]. Data are collected throughout the study and evaluated periodically to determine the efficacy and safety of the drug for the overall population and other points of interest to determine the treatment outcomes [12, 13]. Patients are generally followed for a predetermined, fixed time, such as for 5 years.

Benefits and Limitations of Registry Studies

Benefits of Registry Studies

Registries provide an opportunity to study patient behavior in a real-life setting. During a registry study, data can be organized and evaluated based on many categorical points such as population residence, disease type, age, race, comorbidities, and length of treatment. These data are obtained in a patient's natural environment and more closely represent the patient population than data obtained from RCTs [14]. Populations followed in registries are relatively large compared to RCTs, and data can be used to systematically and prospectively evaluate and monitor long-term safety and AEs for large patient populations [11]. Registry data can be used to confirm previous RCT data, such as the low risk of AEs such as serious infection, defined as an infection requiring hospitalization according to International Classification of Disease-10 (ICD-10) codes. Data can be used for post-marketing surveillance, long-term safety, effectiveness, and long-term outcomes to evaluate drugs in both a prospective and retrospective manner [9, 13, 15–17]. Patient persistence on treatment can also be determined by tracking patient use and cessation of the drugs within the study [18, 19].

Limitations of Registries

Despite the many benefits of registries, there are limitations. Many registries lack established control groups and alternative therapy comparison groups to compare treatment efficacy and safety in similar groups over time, which are often present in an RCT [16]. Participants in registries may be lost to follow-up if they transition to a treatment not followed through the registry, such as topical or nonbiologic systemic therapy [16]. Drug price and supply may change, making it difficult for participants in the registry to obtain these therapies, leading to higher attrition [20]. Terms and definitions for patient populations, regions, and inclusion criteria can vary, limiting the comparison of data in between registries [12]. Patients who enroll voluntarily may differ from those who do not. Registry data are collected based on established treatments, while novel treatment modalities are not typically tracked, as in RCTs, limiting the opportunity to discover new treatment approaches [12].

Because registry subjects are not randomized to different treatment arms, registries share limitations common to other observational studies such as nonresponse bias and confounding bias. Data may be limited due to incomplete reporting of information by the participants or poor data collection methods by the practitioner [16]. If patients have been on multiple treatments over time, it may be difficult to determine which drug is the cause of an AE.

Key Findings from Psoriasis Registry Studies Concerning Biologic Agents

Many registries have been created for biologic therapy for psoriasis. The major psoriasis registries identified as of June 2021 include Corrona Psoriasis Registry (CorEvitas) [21], BADBIR, BIOBADADERM, Continuous Assessment of Psoriasis Treatment Use Registry with Biologics (BioCAPTURE), Swedish Registry for Systemic Psoriasis (PsoReg) [13], PSOLAR, Child-Capture [13], Psocare [13], Psonet [13], Biological Treatment in Danish Dermatology (DERMBIO), Psoriasis Registry Austria (PsoRA), German Psoriasis Registry (PsoBest) [13], Malaysia Psoriasis Registry (MPR) [13], AMC Psoriasis Registry [13], LaCurna Psoriasis Registry [13], Australian Psoriasis Registry [22], Swedish National Psoriasis Register [23], Swiss Registry SDNTT [24], PsoREP [25], PsoBioTeq [25], Clalit Health Service Database [25], Psodit

[25], Psoreal [25], and Swiss Dermatology Network for Biologicals (SDNB) [25]. Registries were identified through systematic analyses and keyword search for "(((psoriasis) AND (registr*)) AND (biologic*)) NOT (clinical trial) NOT (case series)" on PubMED. Registries included were specifically for psoriasis and not for combined rheumatologic diseases, psoriatic arthritis, or pharmaceuticals. Unnamed registries were not included in the final list of major registries. The information was organized in a spreadsheet according to publication, the name of registry, the number of patients enrolled, biologic and nonbiologic treatments, methods, and results.

Long-Term Safety and Tolerability

Biologics have an AE profile like many other drugs, and AEs are evaluated through several methods. Registry data can be used to track long-term safety and tolerability of biologic treatment for psoriasis; registries are listed with their major findings below.

PSOLAR

PSOLAR is a long-term registry sponsored by Janssen Scientific Affairs, LLC for patients with plaque psoriasis exposed to infliximab, ustekinumab, and other biologic or nonbiologic standard-of-care treatments. Patients are followed for up to 8 years [26]. Long-term safety and AEs have been evaluated in multiple studies of data from the PSOLAR registry. Ustekinumab was not associated with an increased risk of serious infections when compared to other biologics and nonbiologic treatments, with an unadjusted serious infection rate of 0.93 per 100 patient-years (PY, defined as the number of AEs per 100 patients per year) [27]. Exposure to infliximab was associated with infection rates of 2.91 per 100 PY, and biologics other than infliximab or ustekinumab were associated with infection rates of 1.91 per 100 PY (no p-values or CI provided). Exposure to infliximab, adalimumab, and etanercept was a predictor for higher rates of serious infection (HR = 1.96, 95% CI: 1.57–2.44, $p < 0.001$) [27].

The rate of serious infection for all patients enrolled in PSOLAR, irrespective of treatment, was 1.45 per 100 PY [10, 28]. The rate of serious infection for each biologic was 0.83 per 100 PY for ustekinumab (CI 0.61–1.09), 1.47 per 100 PY for etanercept (CI 1.10–1.91), 1.97 per 100 PY for adalimumab (CI 1.61–2.39), and 2.49 per 100 PY for infliximab (CI 1.88–3.23) [28]. The rate of serious infection for those not on methotrexate or biologics was 1.05 per 100 PY (CI 0.75–1.43), and the rate of serious infection for those on methotrexate or nonbiologics, but not on a biologic, was 1.28 per 100 PY (0.73–2.09) (no p-value available) [28] Infections included opportunistic infections such as toxoplasmosis, herpes zoster, tuberculosis, and fungal infections, especially candida. The most commonly reported infections occurring in those enrolled in the PSOLAR registry were pneumonia and cellulitis [28]. Serious infection was associated with increasing age, diabetes mellitus, smoking, infection history, infliximab exposure, and adalimumab exposure [28].

The risk of malignancy associated with biologic use in patients enrolled in PSOLAR was 0.61 cases per 100 PY (no p-value available) [10]. Biologics were not associated with increased risk of malignancy, major adverse cardiovascular event (MACE), or mortality (0.68 per 100 PY, 0.33 per 100 PY, and 0.46 per 100 PY, respectively) [27]. Ustekinumab, infliximab, and other biologics were not associated with increased risk of malignancy compared to nonbiologic systemic treatments (0.48 per 100 PY, 0.79 per 100 PY, 0.73 per 100 PY, and 0.84 per 100 PY, respectively) [27]. Patients treated with biologics and registered with PSOLAR had a 0.30 per 100 PY risk of MACE, 0.10 per 100 PY risk of cardiovascular death, 0.08 per 100 PY risk of nonfatal CVA, and 0.13 per 100 PY risk of nonfatal MI, compared to patients on nonbiologic treatments, who had a 0.47 per 100 PY risk of MACE, 0.21 per 100 PY risk of cardiovascular death, 0.10 per 100 PY risk of nonfatal CVA, and 0.19 per 100 PY risk of nonfatal MI [27]. All-cause mortality in a separate study was 0.37 cases per 100 PY, and the rate of cardiovascular events was 0.36 per

100 PY in all patients enrolled in PSOLAR, regardless of treatment [10].

Patients treated with biologics for moderate-to-severe psoriasis had a lower mortality rate regardless of treatment duration (odds ratio [OR] 0.08, CI 0.03–0.23, for less than 1 year; OR 0.08, CI 0.05–0.13 for 1 year or longer). Methotrexate reduced mortality only after 1 year of use (OR 0.18, CI 0.02–1.51 for less than 1 year, OR 0.04, CI 0.01–0.16, for 1 year or longer) [29]. Patients taking adalimumab, etanercept, infliximab, and ustekinumab had no increased risk of cardiovascular event disease [30]. Of 220 women enrolled in the PSOLAR registry who used biologics prenatally, none had an increased risk of pregnancy complications, including spontaneous abortions or congenital abnormalities, compared to the general population (no p-value available) [31].

Psonet

Psonet is a European Registry of Psoriasis for patients treated with either biologic or nonbiologic systemic agents [32]. Multiple studies on long-term biologic agent safety have been completed with Psonet data. Biologics infliximab, adalimumab, and etanercept were not associated with increased serious infection when compared to methotrexate [33]. AEs of biologics should be compared to methotrexate as these therapies are often the only treatments available for severe forms of psoriasis [33]. Risk of first malignancy was not associated with cumulative exposure to infliximab, adalimumab, etanercept, and ustekinumab for inflammatory conditions (OR 1.02, 95% CI 0.92–1.13) [34].

DERMBIO

DERMBIO is a Danish registry for patients with psoriasis receiving biological treatment [35]. Infection was the most common AE associated with adalimumab, etanercept, infliximab, and ustekinumab (17.4 per 100 PY, CI 16.1–18.7; 13.6 per 100 PY, CI 11.8–15.7; 12.1 per 100 PY, CI 9.8–14.9; and 11.6 per 100 PY, CI 11.6–14.4, respectively). Other AEs associated with treatment included nonmelanoma skin cancer, cardiovascular events, neurological events, and other unspecified events [36]. Two cases of inflammatory bowel disease were reported, one with adalimumab and one with infliximab, for a total of 0.01% of all AEs [36].

Persistence on Therapy

Drug survival, also referred to as drug retention or drug persistence, is the length of treatment adherence [19]. Drug persistence may also be defined as the length of time from initiation of therapy to discontinuation. Real-life drug survival for biologics can be determined from large registry studies. Persistence can be measured based on the number of days between refills of the medication [37].

PSOLAR

In the PSOLAR registry, ustekinumab was associated with longer persistence and lower discontinuation compared to adalimumab, etanercept, and infliximab (hazard ratio [HR] 4.99, CI 3.39–7.35, $p < 0.0001$; HR 5.59, CI: 3.77–8.29, $p < 0.0001$; and HR 3.04, CI: 1.66–5.57, $p = 0.0003$, respectively) [38].

BADBIR

BADBIR is a British register for patients with psoriasis treated with biologics and immunomodulators to assess long-term safety of biologic treatments [39]. Patients who would have been eligible for clinical trials were compared to those who would be ineligible compared in the BADBIR registry. Drug discontinuation rates were similar between both cohorts. The most common reason for discontinuation was ineffectiveness (etanercept, 11–15%; adalimumab 6–8%; and ustekinumab 3–5%), followed by AEs (etanercept, 2–4%; adalimumab, 3–5%; ustekinumab, 2–3%) [40]. Female gender, being a current smoker, and having a higher baseline Dermatology Life Quality Index (DLQI) were more likely to discontinue biologic treatment. Patients with psoriatic arthritis were more likely to have longer drug survival. Ustekinumab had the longest first-course drug survival followed by adalimumab. Etanercept and infliximab had the shortest drug survival. After accounting for relevant covariates, ustekinumab had the highest first-course drug survival of the drugs included in the study [41].

DERMBIO

Ustekinumab had higher drug survival than secukinumab, etanercept, and infliximab, which all had similar survival rates in patients registered with DERMBIO. Drug survival was higher in patients who were biologic-naive before treatment than those who failed initial biologic therapy (no p-value available) [36]. Similarly, in a study by Gniadecki et al., ustekinumab had greater drug survival than other TNF-α inhibitors ($p < 0.001$). Etanercept had the shortest drug survival at a median survival of 30 months; adalimumab and infliximab had similar drug survival rates at 59 months and 47 months (CI 25.1–34.9, $p < 0.01$; CI 45.6–72.4, $p < 0.001$; and CI 45.6–72.4, $p = 0.008$, respectively). Survival was longer in men than women and in biologic-naive patients than patients who had previously taken a biologic (OR 1.51, 95% CI 1.31–1.74; OR 1.24, 95% CI 1.05–1.46, respectively). A majority, 67%, of all drug discontinuations were attributed to loss of efficacy [42].

PsoRA

PsoRA is an Austrian registry for patients with psoriasis [43]. Ustekinumab had better drug survival at 48 months than ixekizumab, secukinumab, adalimumab, and etanercept. However, when adjusted for biologic naïveté, ustekinumab had similar drug survival rates to ixekizumab and secukinumab (92.8%, 91.6%, and 90.2%, respectively); all were superior to adalimumab and etanercept at 12 months and later (76.5% and 71.9%, respectively) [44]. Biologic drug survival at 36 months was 51.6% for adalimumab, 56.0% for etanercept, and 22.6% for infliximab ($p = 0.0000007$). Median drug survival was 1264 days for adalimumab (CI 800-infinity), 1438 days for etanercept (CI 1141–1825), and 477 days for infliximab (CI 337–642) [45]. Drug discontinuation was attributed to ineffectiveness, loss of initial response, AEs (most frequently infection), switching to another biologic agent, and/or complete remission [45].

BIOBADADERM

BIOBADADERM is a Spanish registry for patients with psoriasis treated with biologics and other systemic therapies, and follows patients for up to 5 years [46]. In one study of BIOBADADERM Data, the primary reason for discontinuation of biologics based on physician judgment was lack of efficacy followed by remission (36.4% and 27.2%, respectively). Biologics had higher drug survival than older nonbiologic drugs. Ustekinumab had longer drug survival compared to adalimumab, infliximab, and etanercept (79.4 months versus 64.6 months, 63.6 months, and 55.5 months, respectively) [47].

Real-World Efficacy Studies for Psoriasis Biologics

Measuring Efficacy of Treatment

Psoriasis treatment is evaluated with a variety of assessment tools [4]. The PASI measures overall psoriasis lesion severity (erythema, induration, and scaling) and extent of body coverage or body surface area (BSA) [4]. PASI is calculated before, during, and after treatment to determine response to treatment; a decrease in PASI score indicates treatment efficacy [4]. The majority of clinical trials compare biologics to placebo, making it difficult to compare biologics to older nonbiologic systemic treatments [4]. A 75% improvement in the PASI score (PASI 75) is a standard benchmark used to document effectiveness in clinical trials [4]; however, PASI improvement scores of 50, 90, and 100% can also be measured and reported. PASI scoring is generally done only in research settings [48, 49]. PASI is challenging to calculate and interpret and is insensitive to measuring change in mild psoriasis, making it less practical for everyday use [50]. PASI is not tightly correlated with patient perception of disease severity, though they are related [42]. Improvements in objective PASI and subjective quality of life (such as the Dermatology Life Quality Index [DLQI]) scores do correlate in patients with chronic moderate-to-severe psoriasis when treated with biologics. Patients who have a PASI75 success also tend to have considerable improvement in quality of life [51]. The Physician Global Assessment and Body Surface Area composite tool is the product of both (PGA x BSA) and can be used as an outcome measure for psoriasis improvement as an alternative to PASI [50]. The physician assigns an estimate of the overall disease severity with a 7-point scale from clear to severe [4]. BSA can be approximated with 1% of BSA approximately equal to a patient's handprint [4].

Real-World Efficacy of Psoriasis Biologics

Data from multiple psoriasis registries have been analyzed to determine the real-world efficacy of treatment.

PSOLAR

At 6 months, 52.2%, 35.6%, 40.4%, and 40.0% of patients in PSOLAR had ≥ a 2-point reduction in PGA on ustekinumab, infliximab, adalimumab, and etanercept, respectively. At 12 months, 55.3% and 40.0% of patients on ustekinumab and infliximab, respectively, had ≥ a 2-point reduction in PGA (no p-value provided) [52].

BioCAPTURE

BioCAPTURE is a Dutch registry for patients with psoriasis treated with biologics from a network of 17 Dutch hospitals [53]. In a BioCAPTURE study, adalimumab, etanercept, and ustekinumab had similar effectiveness after 1 year of treatment; ustekinumab had the highest effectiveness of the three during 5 years of treatment ($p = 0.047$; ustekinumab versus etanercept, $p = 0.019$). There was a higher chance of attaining PASI 75 with adalimumab and ustekinumab than with etanercept at 1 year of treatment [54].

PsoRA

Adalimumab and infliximab had better short-term effectiveness than etanercept in a PsoRA study. PASI 75 was achieved in 65% of adalimumab, 49.7% of etanercept, and 69.8% of infliximab cycles at 4 months. PASI 90 was achieved in 35.7% of adalimumab, 21.2% of etanercept, and 50.9% of infliximab cycles at 4 months (no *p*-value provided) [45].

DERMBIO

Secukinumab had the fastest onset of action and highest number of PASI 100 respondents when compared with adalimumab, etanercept, infliximab, and ustekinumab. Secukinumab also had the highest proportion of patients achieving a PASI of ≤2 or ≤1, respectively (but not ≤5), among bio-naïve patients [36].

Conclusion

Biologics improve outcomes and minimize disease burden in patients suffering from psoriasis. Registries are powerful tools that further the understanding of the benefit of biologic therapy compared to nonbiologic therapy in the treatment of psoriasis. Registry data collected on place of residence, disease type, age, race, and comorbidities may help identify factors that predict treatment response. Registry data on dosing, length of treatment, refills, patient outcomes, and patient well-being over time demonstrate the benefit of biologics and the increased overall effectiveness and better safety profile compared to older systemic therapies. Registry data on long-term safety and overall effectiveness confirm the benefits seen in RCTs in a real-world environment that is more representative of the broader population.

Biologics have better overall drug survival compared to older small molecule systemic drugs. However, drug survival on biologics is lower in patients previously treated with a biologic compared to drug survival in patients with no previous biologic treatment. The increased drug survival of biologics compared to older systemic therapies may partly be due to the greater efficacy, fewer side effects, or possibly dosing schedules that include a longer interval between medication administration, leading to greater adherence and more prolonged use.

Comparisons can be made within and between biologic classes. Ustekinumab has better drug survival than TNF-α inhibitors, while etanercept had the lowest drug survival. Additionally, ustekinumab was least frequently associated with discontinuation due to loss of efficacy and had the lowest 1-year and 2-year cost per PASI 75 responder [19]. These characteristics may contribute to the increased drug survival of ustekinumab. Etanercept, however, was associated with the greatest discontinuation due to loss of efficacy and greater injection site reactions [19]. Regular blood tests are required for its use, which may contribute to its lower drug survival rates [55]. Overall, the most common reason for discontinuation of biologics across many studies was perceived lack of efficacy and disease remission [40–42, 47].

Registries can be used to approximate drug efficacy in real-life situations. Efficacy can be measured using PASI and PGA scores. Secukinumab had higher efficacy than ustekinumab, adalimumab, and etanercept in registries, confirming what was expected from RCT data. The newest IL-17A and IL-23 blocking drugs appear to be more effective than older biologic treatments [56].

Psoriasis registry data can be used to study AEs associated with biologic treatment compared to older systemic treatments, providing critical information about biologic safety in real-life use in broader populations (including those with comorbidities) than are treated in clinical trials. AEs occur at lower rates within biologics compared to older systemic psoriasis medications. AE rates in patients on biologics appear comparable, perhaps even lower, than in patients not on any systemic treatment for their psoriasis.

In conjunction with RCTs, registries have been used to understand biologics' long-term treatment efficacy, safety, AEs, adherence, and drug survival. This information can assist physicians and patients to make informed decisions about psoriasis treatment options, ultimately leading to better patient outcomes.

Disclosures Dr. Steven Feldman has received research, speaking, and/or consulting support from a variety of companies including Galderma, GSK/Stiefel, Almirall, Leo Pharma, Boehringer Ingelheim, Mylan, Celgene, Pfizer, Valeant, AbbVie, Samsung, Janssen, Lilly, Menlo, Merck, Novartis, Regeneron, Sanofi, Novan, Qurient, National Biological Corporation, Caremark, Advance Medical, Sun Pharma, Suncare Research, Informa, UpToDate, and National Psoriasis Foundation. He is founder and majority owner of www.DrScore.com and founder and part owner of Causa Research, a company dedicated to enhancing patients' adherence to treatment. Mrs. Cull, Mr. Pena, Dr. Balogh, and Ms. Purvis have no conflicts to disclose.

References

1. Alexander GC, Ogasawara K, Wiegand D, Lin D, Breder CD. Clinical development of biologics approved by the US Food and Drug Administration, 2003-2016. Ther Innov Regul Sci. 2019;53(6):752–8. https://doi.org/10.1177/2168479018812058.
2. Rich SJ, Bello-Quintero CE. Advancements in the treatment of psoriasis: role of biologic agents. J Manag Care Pharm. 2004;10(4):318–25. https://doi.org/10.18553/jmcp.2004.10.4.318.
3. Armstrong AW, Read C. Pathophysiology, clinical presentation, and treatment of psoriasis: a review. JAMA. 2020;323(19):1945–60. https://doi.org/10.1001/jama.2020.4006.
4. Menter A, Gottlieb A, Feldman SR, Van Voorhees AS, Leonardi CL, Gordon KB, et al. Guidelines of care for the management of psoriasis and psoriatic arthritis: section 1. Overview of psoriasis and guidelines of care for the treatment of psoriasis with biologics. J Am Acad Dermatol. 2008;58(5):826–50. https://doi.org/10.1016/j.jaad.2008.02.039.
5. Rendon A, Schakel K. Psoriasis pathogenesis and treatment. Int J Mol Sci. 2019;20(6) https://doi.org/10.3390/ijms20061475.
6. Kim WB, Marinas JE, Qiang J, Shahbaz A, Greaves S, Yeung J. Adverse events resulting in withdrawal of biologic therapy for psoriasis in real-world clinical practice: a Canadian multicenter retrospective study. J Am Acad Dermatol. 2015;73(2):237–41. https://doi.org/10.1016/j.jaad.2015.04.023.
7. Papp KA, Dekoven J, Parsons L, Pirzada S, Robern M, Robertson L, et al. Biologic therapy in psoriasis: perspectives on associated risks and patient management. J Cutan Med Surg. 2012;16(3):153–68. https://doi.org/10.1177/120347541201600305.
8. McCambridge J, Witton J, Elbourne DR. Systematic review of the Hawthorne effect: new concepts are needed to study research participation effects. J Clin Epidemiol. 2014;67(3):267–77. https://doi.org/10.1016/j.jclinepi.2013.08.015.
9. Registries – DSRU. 2021. https://www.dsru.org/service/registries/ Accessed 18 Apr 2021.
10. Papp KA, Strober B, Augustin M, Calabro S, Londhe A, Chevrier M, et al. PSOLAR: design, utility, and preliminary results of a prospective, international,

disease-based registry of patients with psoriasis who are receiving, or are candidates for, conventional systemic treatments or biologic agents. J Drugs Dermatol. 2012;11(10):1210–7.
11. Burden AD, Warren RB, Kleyn CE, McElhone K, Smith CH, Reynolds NJ, et al. The British Association of Dermatologists' Biologic Interventions Register (BADBIR): design, methodology and objectives. Br J Dermatol. 2012;166(3):545–54. https://doi.org/10.1111/j.1365-2133.2012.10835.x.
12. Janssen Scientific Affairs L: Psoriasis Longitudinal Assessment and Registry (PSOLAR). 2021. https://clinicaltrials.gov/ct2/show/NCT00508547 (2007). Accessed 18 Apr 2021.
13. Eissing L, Rustenbach SJ, Krensel M, Zander N, Spehr C, Radtke MA, et al. Psoriasis registries worldwide: systematic overview on registry publications. J Eur Acad Dermatol Venereol. 2016;30(7):1100–6. https://doi.org/10.1111/jdv.13634.
14. Lecluse LL, Naldi L, Stern RS, Spuls PI. National registries of systemic treatment for psoriasis and the European 'Psonet' initiative. Dermatology. 2009;218(4):347–56. https://doi.org/10.1159/000183757.
15. Amin M, Lee EB, Bhutani T, Wu JJ. Review of European registries for psoriasis. J Dermatolog Treat. 2019;30(3):227–36. https://doi.org/10.1080/09546634.2018.1506084.
16. Amin M, No DJ, Wu JJ. Review of U.S. registries for psoriasis. J Dermatolog Treat. 2017;28(8):697–701. https://doi.org/10.1080/09546634.2017.1328549.
17. DiMarco G, Hill D, Feldman SR. Review of patient registries in dermatology. J Am Acad Dermatol. 2016;75(4):824–9. https://doi.org/10.1016/j.jaad.2016.03.020.
18. Geale K, Lindberg I, Paulsson EC, Wennerstrom ECM, Tjarnlund A, Noel W, et al. Persistence of biologic treatments in psoriatic arthritis: a population-based study in Sweden. Rheumatol Adv Pract. 2020;4(2):rkaa070. https://doi.org/10.1093/rap/rkaa070.
19. Lin PT, Wang SH, Chi CC. Drug survival of biologics in treating psoriasis: a meta-analysis of real-world evidence. Sci Rep. 2018;8(1):16068. https://doi.org/10.1038/s41598-018-34293-y.
20. Heymann W. The newest frontier for biologics and psoriasis may be adherence. Rosemont: The American Academy of Dermatology Association; 2019.
21. The Corrona Psoriasis (PSO) Registry. https://clinicaltrials.gov/ct2/show/NCT02707341 Accessed 2021.
22. Doolan BJ, Koye D, Ling J, Cains GD, Baker C, Foley P, et al. Treatment modalities and risk of adverse events associated with biologic therapy: a 10-year observational review of the Australasian Psoriasis Registry. Australas J Dermatol. 2021;62(1):e47–54. https://doi.org/10.1111/ajd.13450.
23. Hjalte F, Carlsson KS, Schmitt-Egenolf M. Sustained Psoriasis Area and Severity Index, Dermatology Life Quality Index and EuroQol-5D response of biological treatment in psoriasis: 10 years of real-world data in the Swedish National Psoriasis Register. Br J Dermatol. 2018;178(1):245–52. https://doi.org/10.1111/bjd.15757.
24. Maul JT, Djamei V, Kolios AGA, Meier B, Czernielewski J, Jungo P, et al. Efficacy and survival of systemic psoriasis treatments: an analysis of the Swiss Registry SDNTT. Dermatology. 2016;232(6):640–7. https://doi.org/10.1159/000452740.
25. Naldi L. Infections and psoriasis treatment: more "real-world" data needed with critical appraisal. J Invest Dermatol. 2017;137(2):271–4. https://doi.org/10.1016/j.jid.2016.10.022.
26. Psoriasis Longitudinal Assessment and Registry – full text view – ClinicalTrials.gov. 2021. https://clinicaltrials.gov/ct2/show/NCT00508547. Accessed 25 July 2021.
27. Papp K, Gottlieb AB, Naldi L, Pariser D, Ho V, Goyal K, et al. Safety surveillance for ustekinumab and other psoriasis treatments from the Psoriasis Longitudinal Assessment and Registry (PSOLAR). J Drugs Dermatol. 2015;14(7):706–14.
28. Kalb RE, Fiorentino DF, Lebwohl MG, Toole J, Poulin Y, Cohen AD, et al. Risk of serious infection with biologic and systemic treatment of psoriasis results from the Psoriasis Longitudinal Assessment and Registry (PSOLAR). JAMA Dermatol. 2015;151(9):961–9. https://doi.org/10.1001/jamadermatol.2015.0718.
29. Langley RG, Poulin Y, Srivastava B, Lafferty KP, Fakharzadeh S, Langholff W, et al. Reduced risk of mortality associated with systemic psoriasis treatment in the Psoriasis Longitudinal Assessment and Registry (PSOLAR): a nested case-control analysis. J Am Acad Dermatol. 2021;84(1):60–9. https://doi.org/10.1016/j.jaad.2020.08.032.
30. PSOLAR results show no patterns of cardiovascular events. 2014. https://www.dermatologytimes.com/view/psolar-results-show-no-patterns-cardiovascular-events. Accessed May 9, 2021.
31. Kimball AB, Guenther L, Kalia S, de Jong E, Lafferty KP, Chen DY, et al. Pregnancy outcomes in women with moderate-to-severe psoriasis from the Psoriasis Longitudinal Assessment and Registry (PSOLAR). JAMA Dermatol. 2021;157(3):301–6. https://doi.org/10.1001/jamadermatol.2020.5595.
32. PSONET: European Registry of Psoriasis. http://www.psonet.eu/cms/ 2021. Accessed July 1, 2021.
33. Garcia-Doval I, Cohen AD, Cazzaniga S, Feldhamer I, Addis A, Carretero G, et al. Risk of serious infections, cutaneous bacterial infections, and granulomatous infections in patients with psoriasis treated with anti-tumor necrosis factor agents versus classic therapies: prospective meta-analysis of Psonet registries. J Am Acad Dermatol. 2017;76(2):299–308 e16. https://doi.org/10.1016/j.jaad.2016.07.039.
34. Garcia-Doval I, Descalzo MA, Mason KJ, Cohen AD, Ormerod AD, Gomez-Garcia FJ, et al. Cumulative exposure to biological therapy and risk of cancer in patients with psoriasis: a meta-analysis of Psonet stud-

ies from Israel, Italy, Spain, the U.K. and Republic of Ireland. Br J Dermatol. 2018;179(4):863–71. https://doi.org/10.1111/bjd.16715.
35. Biological treatment in Danish dermatology. https://www.danishhealthdata.com/find-health-data/National-kvalitetsdatabase-for-psoriasispatienter-i-biologisk-behandling. Accessed 25 July 2021.
36. Egeberg A, Ottosen MB, Gniadecki R, Broesby-Olsen S, Dam TN, Bryld LE, et al. Safety, efficacy and drug survival of biologics and biosimilars for moderate-to-severe plaque psoriasis. Br J Dermatol. 2018;178(2):509–19. https://doi.org/10.1111/bjd.16102.
37. Cramer JA, Roy A, Burrell A, Fairchild CJ, Fuldeore MJ, Ollendorf DA, et al. Medication compliance and persistence: terminology and definitions. Value Health. 2008;11(1):44–7. https://doi.org/10.1111/j.1524-4733.2007.00213.x.
38. New findings from the Psoriasis Longitudinal Assessment And Registry (PSOLAR) show persistency difference among biologic therapies | Johnson & Johnson.
39. BADBIR – study information. 2021. http://www.badbir.org/Clinicians/Information/StudyInformation/ Accessed 25 July 2021.
40. Mason KJ, Barker J, Smith CH, Hampton PJ, Lunt M, McElhone K, et al. Comparison of drug discontinuation, effectiveness, and safety between clinical trial eligible and ineligible patients in BADBIR. JAMA Dermatol. 2018;154(5):581–8. https://doi.org/10.1001/jamadermatol.2018.0183.
41. Warren RB, Smith CH, Yiu ZZN, Ashcroft DM, Barker J, Burden AD, et al. Differential drug survival of biologic therapies for the treatment of psoriasis: a prospective observational cohort study from the British Association of Dermatologists Biologic Interventions Register (BADBIR). J Invest Dermatol. 2015;135(11):2632–40. https://doi.org/10.1038/jid.2015.208.
42. Gniadecki R, Bang B, Bryld LE, Iversen L, Lasthein S, Skov L. Comparison of long-term drug survival and safety of biologic agents in patients with psoriasis vulgaris. Br J Dermatol. 2015;172(1):244–52. https://doi.org/10.1111/bjd.13343.
43. PsoRA. https://psora.medunigraz.at/en/ Accessed 25 July 2021.
44. Graier T, Salmhofer W, Jonak C, Weger W, Kolli C, Gruber B, et al. Biologic drug survival rates in the era of anti-Il-17 antibodies: a time period-adjusted registry analysis. Br J Dermatol. 2020; https://doi.org/10.1111/bjd.19701.
45. Inzinger M, Wippel-Slupetzky K, Weger W, Richter L, Mlynek A, Fleischander B, et al. Survival and effectiveness of tumour necrosis factor-alpha inhibitors in the treatment of plaque psoriasis under daily life conditions: report from the Psoriasis Registry Austria. Acta Derm Venereol. 2016;96(2):207–12. https://doi.org/10.2340/00015555-2214.
46. Spanish Registry of Systemic Treatments in Psoriasis – full text view – ClinicalTrials.gov. 2021. https://clinicaltrials.gov/ct2/show/NCT02075697 Accessed 25 July 2021.
47. Davila-Seijo P, Dauden E, Carretero G, Ferrandiz C, Vanaclocha F, Gomez-Garcia FJ, et al. Survival of classic and biological systemic drugs in psoriasis: results of the BIOBADADERM registry and critical analysis. J Eur Acad Dermatol Venereol. 2016;30(11):1942–50. https://doi.org/10.1111/jdv.13682.
48. Clinical review report: Guselkumab (Tremfya): (Janssen Inc): indication: for the treatment of adult patients with moderate-to-severe plaque psoriasis who are candidates for systemic therapy or phototherapy. CADTH Common Drug Reviews. Ottawa (ON) 2018.
49. Belinchon Romero I, Dauden E, Ferrandiz Foraster C, Gonzalez-Cantero A, Carrascosa Carrillo JM, Psoriasis Group of the Spanish Academy of Dermatology and Venereology, et al. PASI 100 response rates in moderate to severe psoriasis: a systematic literature review and analysis of clinical practice guidelines. J Dermatolog Treat. 2021:1–9. https://doi.org/10.1080/09546634.2021.1890683.
50. Walsh JA, Jones H, Mallbris L, Duffin KC, Krueger GG, Clegg DO, et al. The physician global assessment and body surface area composite tool is a simple alternative to the Psoriasis Area and Severity Index for assessment of psoriasis: post hoc analysis from PRISTINE and PRESTA. Psoriasis (Auckl). 2018;8:65–74. https://doi.org/10.2147/PTT.S169333.
51. Mattei PL, Corey KC, Kimball AB. Psoriasis Area Severity Index (PASI) and the Dermatology Life Quality Index (DLQI): the correlation between disease severity and psychological burden in patients treated with biological therapies. J Eur Acad Dermatol Venereol. 2014;28(3):333–7. https://doi.org/10.1111/jdv.12106.
52. Strober BE, Bissonnette R, Fiorentino D, Kimball AB, Naldi L, Shear NH, et al. Comparative effectiveness of biologic agents for the treatment of psoriasis in a real-world setting: results from a large, prospective, observational study (Psoriasis Longitudinal Assessment and Registry [PSOLAR]). J Am Acad Dermatol. 2016;74(5):851–61 e4. https://doi.org/10.1016/j.jaad.2015.12.017.
53. What is BioCAPTURE – Het BioCAPTURE onderzoek. 2021. https://biocapture.nl/?lang=en Accessed 25 July 2021.
54. Zweegers J, Groenewoud JMM, van den Reek J, Otero ME, van de Kerkhof PCM, Driessen RJB, et al. Comparison of the 1- and 5-year effectiveness of adalimumab, etanercept and ustekinumab in patients with psoriasis in daily clinical practice: results from the prospective BioCAPTURE registry. Br J Dermatol. 2017;176(4):1001–9. https://doi.org/10.1111/bjd.15023.
55. Compare Enbrel vs. Stelara. 2021. https://www.iodine.com/compare/enbrel-vs-stelara. Accessed 1 July 2021.
56. von Stebut E, Boehncke WH, Ghoreschi K, Gori T, Kaya Z, Thaci D, et al. IL-17A in psoriasis and beyond: cardiovascular and metabolic implications. Front Immunol. 2019;10:3096. https://doi.org/10.3389/fimmu.2019.03096.

Psoriasis Biologic Agents in Special Populations

11

Akshitha Thatiparthi, Amylee Martin, Jeffrey Liu, George Han, and Jashin J. Wu

Abbreviations

CD4+	Cluster of differentiation 4
CI	Confidence interval
FC	Fragment, crystallizable
FDA	Food and Drug Administration
HIV	Human immunodeficiency virus
IL	Interleukin
NMSC	Nonmelanoma skin cancer
NPF	National Psoriasis Foundation
OR	Odds ratio
PASI	Psoriasis Area and Severity Index
PGA	Physician Global Assessment and Body Surface Area

A. Thatiparthi
College of Osteopathic Medicine of the Pacific, Western University of Health Sciences, Pomona, CA, USA

A. Martin
School of Medicine, University of California, Riverside, CA, USA

J. Liu
Keck School of Medicine, University of Southern California, Los Angeles, CA, USA

G. Han
Icahn School of Medicine at Mount Sinai, New York City, NY, USA

J. J. Wu (✉)
Dermatology Research and Education Foundation, Irvine, CA, USA

Introduction

Plaque psoriasis is an inflammatory skin condition with features of autoimmunity. The first biologic was approved for the treatment of psoriasis in 2003 [1]. Improved understanding of the pathogenesis of psoriasis has allowed for the development and approval of 11 biologics thus far, with several more in the pipeline [2]. However, increased availability of therapeutic options can make selection of an optimal biologic challenging for patients and physicians. Patients who are pregnant, have human immunodeficiency virus (HIV), have a history of nonmelanoma skin cancer (NMSC)/lymphoma, are elderly, or are undergoing surgery may be excluded from clinical trials, resulting in insufficient data on biologic safety and efficacy in these populations. In this chapter, we provide evidence-based algorithms for Food and Drug Administration (FDA)-approved biologics in the treatment of moderate-to-severe psoriasis for special populations. Additionally, an upcoming precision medicine tool using psoriasis, biomarkers, and patient RNA will be highlighted.

Approved biologics for the treatment of moderate-to-severe psoriasis include the following [3, 4]:

N. Brownstone et al. (eds.), *Biologic Therapy for Psoriasis*, Updates in Clinical Dermatology,
https://doi.org/10.1007/978-3-030-92938-1_11

- Tumor necrosis factor (TNF)-alpha inhibitors: infliximab, etanercept, adalimumab, and certolizumab
- Interleukin (IL)-12/23 inhibitor: ustekinumab
- IL-17 inhibitors: secukinumab, ixekizumab, and brodalumab
- IL-23p19 inhibitors: guselkumab, tildrakizumab, and risankizumab.

Biologics for Pregnant and Breastfeeding Patients

Treating moderate-to-severe psoriasis in patients who are pregnant or breastfeeding poses some complexity in therapeutics and management. While some patients report clinical improvement of psoriasis during pregnancy, others describe worsening of symptoms and require systemic therapies for disease management [5]. As clinical trials often exclude pregnant and breastfeeding patients due to neonatal and infant risk, data on biologic use are limited, especially in humans [6].

Certolizumab is reported to be safe for use during pregnancy and breastfeeding due to the lack of a fragment, crystallizable (Fc) region. The absence of this domain prevents active placental transfer during pregnancy and lactation [7]. Analysis of safety outcomes for 528 patients with chronic inflammatory conditions exposed to certolizumab during pregnancy did not report an increased teratogenic risk or fetal demise compared to the general population [8]. In a prospective pharmacokinetic study (n = 14) of certolizumab treatment for inflammatory conditions during pregnancy, all infants had minimal (n = 1) to no (n = 13) transfer of certolizumab at birth and no quantifiable levels of certolizumab after 8 weeks [7]. Further, a pharmacokinetic study of 17 patients demonstrated zero to minimal transfer of certolizumab during breastfeeding [9]. Thus, certolizumab is a safe and efficacious drug for this group.

In general, it is important to keep in mind that biologics do not cross the placenta in appreciable amounts in the first and most of the second trimester [10]. As such, in general, a decision on biologic treatment does not have to be made until after the pregnancy is confirmed. In a large study analyzing 2,220,332 patients treated with TNF-alpha inhibitors during pregnancy, a subcohort of 6791 patients had a history of psoriasis [11]. The study reported a preference for treatment with etanercept in the first trimester [11]. After the first trimester, TNF-alpha inhibitor usage decreased except for certolizumab and infliximab [11]. In another population-based study of pregnancy and birth outcomes in chronic inflammatory skin conditions, 1027 patients treated with TNF-alpha inhibitors (infliximab, etanercept, and adalimumab) were compared to 9399 patients treated with nonsystemic biologics [12]. The study reported a higher risk of preterm births and intrauterine growth restriction with exposure to infliximab compared to adalimumab and etanercept [12]. Additionally, a case series of seven women with 10 pregnancies treated with infliximab, adalimumab, or ustekinumab reported that the pregnant patients did not experience any adverse events with treatment and none of the babies were born with congenital anomalies [13]. Caution is recommended with live vaccinations for infants due to risk of infection with the use of TNF-alpha inhibitors in pregnancy [11].

According to the FDA, ustekinumab and secukinumab were classified as pregnancy category B in the previous pregnancy category system. With regard to real-world experience, a case series of 10 pregnancies (involving 7 mothers) with exposure to ustekinumab did not report adverse events for the mothers or infants. Notably, ustekinumab was discontinued in the first trimester in 9 pregnancies and in the third trimester in 1 pregnancy [14]. Additional case reports have supported similar findings for ustekinumab exposure in pregnancy and infants [15–18]. Information on breastfeeding with ustekinumab is sparse; however, the drug is hypothesized to be safe due to the large molecule size [19]. In an analysis of pooled pregnancy data from two studies (n = 292), rates of spontaneous abortion and congenital anomalies were comparable to the general population [20]. Given that secukinumab may cross the placental barrier later in pregnancy, most patients discontinued treatment in the first trimester [20]. Further, the benefits and risks of secukinumab should be discussed with the patients before utilizing the agent in pregnancy and/or breastfeeding.

Limited studies exist regarding the study of ixekizumab, brodalumab, and IL-23 inhibitors in pregnancy, with available data being limited to animal studies in pregnant monkeys [21–25]. As ixekizumab, brodalumab, tildrakizumab, risankizumab, and guselkumab are monoclonal IgG antibodies, these biologics can cross the placenta and be excreted in breast milk during lactation, which needs to be taken into consideration for humans in pregnancy and breastfeeding [21–25].

Expert opinion algorithm:

1. Certolizumab
2. Etanercept
3. Ustekinumab or secukinumab (class B with old pregnancy classes)
4. Adalimumab or infliximab
5. Ixekizumab, brodalumab, and IL-23 inhibitors.

Biologics for Patients Who Are HIV-Positive

HIV was reported to affect 37.9 million people worldwide in 2018 [26]. The severity of chronic HIV has been noted to be positively correlated with the severity of psoriasis [27]. Additionally, HIV may induce psoriasis flares in patients with pre-existing disease. The chronic immunosuppressive state presents a therapeutic challenge as systemic immunomodulator treatments, such as biologics, can further suppress the immune system. Given that psoriasis is a T-cell-mediated disease and HIV depletes T cells [27], it has been a bit of a conundrum to ascertain why psoriasis can flare in patients with HIV and this entity has helped to elucidate critical inflammatory pathways in psoriasis itself [28]. Overall, patients with HIV and psoriasis require regular follow-up with a multidisciplinary approach involving dermatologists and infectious disease specialists [29].

TNF-alpha inhibitors and ustekinumab should be utilized with caution in patients with concomitant HIV and psoriasis. Patients require monitoring of cluster of differentiation 4 (CD4+) T-cell count/HIV viral load, must demonstrate no recent history of opportunistic infections, and receive highly active antiretroviral therapy to be considered for therapy [27, 30]. Prior to initiating TNF-alpha inhibitor therapy, patients should be screened for HIV [31]. If the HIV test is positive and the CD4+ count is less than 200 in a HIV-positive patient with psoriasis, TNF-alpha inhibitor therapy should not initiate [31]. In a case report of a 45-year-old man with psoriasis, psoriatic arthritis, and HIV, the patient had improvement of psoriasis and psoriatic arthritis, while HIV viral load and CD4+ cell count remained stable through 4 months of etanercept treatment [32]. However, the patient had to discontinue etanercept due to the development of polymicrobial infections [32]. Three other case reports ($n = 4$) showed positive psoriasis clinical outcomes in patients with HIV treated with etanercept, with one patient treated for 6 years and other patients not having notable side effects [33–35]. Additionally, case reports have showed treatment efficacy for ustekinumab ($n = 2$) and adalimumab ($n = 1$) in HIV+ psoriasis patients [36–38]. A multicenter study ($n = 23$) of HIV-positive patients with psoriasis treated with etanercept, ustekinumab, or methotrexate showed treatment efficacy and an acceptable safety profile for TNF-alpha inhibitors and ustekinumab [39]. Another case series had similar findings in four patients receiving ustekinumab and six patients receiving TNF-alpha inhibitors, with all 100 achieving psoriasis area and severity index (PASI) 75 with stable CD4+ counts [40]. A PubMed search was performed on July 18, 2021, for literature on certolizumab treatment in HIV+ patients with psoriasis, and no studies were identified. However, the FDA-prescribing information states patients with HIV exposed to certolizumab have a higher risk of infections [41].

Two recent case reports have shown effective treatment of psoriasis with IL-17 inhibitors, with one patient experiencing candida esophagitis [42, 43]. There are no published reports for other IL-17 inhibitors and for IL-23 inhibitors in this psoriasis patient population.

It is good practice to consider evaluating HIV seropositivity status prior to the initiation of treatment with biologics in many patients. If the patient is HIV-positive, highly active antiretroviral therapy is indicated along with regular monitoring of viral load and CD4+ count by infectious disease specialists and dermatologists. As TNF-alpha inhibitors and ustekinumab have shown efficacy and relatively favorable safety profiles, these two classes are first line for this population. As research for IL-17 inhibitors and Il-23 inhibitors is limited, they are lower in terms of preference in our algorithm, although there is no theoretical evidence that there should be any additional safety signals with these classes of medications.

Expert opinion algorithm:

1. TNF-alpha inhibitors or ustekinumab
   - Receiving highly active antiretroviral therapy (HAART)
   - Normal CD4+ T-cell count
   - No recent history of opportunistic infections
2. IL-17 inhibitors or IL-23 inhibitors

Biologics for Patients with History of Malignancy (NMSC and Lymphoma)

Due to the chronic inflammatory state of psoriasis and immunosuppression induced by some systemic agents, patients with psoriasis have an increased risk of lymphoma and NMSC [44–48]. Patients receiving biologic therapy should be routinely screened for age-appropriate routine malignancies including breast, cervical, colon, and lung cancer [46].

Pooled data from multiple phase II and III clinical trials with long-term safety data through 5 years for ustekinumab in the treatment of psoriasis reported the risk of malignancy to be negligible [49–51]. However, there was a recent case report of a female receiving ustekinumab also developing stage IV Hodgkin lymphoma, raising concern for oncogenic potential [52]. While the majority of data and clinical experience with ustekinumab suggest that there are no major issues with malignancy and IL-12/23 inhibition, there is evidence that IL-12 functions in an antitumor fashion, and thus, blocking IL-12 would not be preferable from a theoretical standpoint [53]. However, longitudinal safety data (n = 12,093) evaluating biologics, including ustekinumab, do not support this concern as the data analysis did not demonstrate an increased risk for malignancy in patients treated with ustekinumab [54].

The effect of IL-17 inhibitor use on malignancy development/progression remains unclear due to the pro-tumorigenic and antitumorigenic potential of IL-17 [55]. However, a pooled analysis of ten phase II and phase III clinical trials reported zero cases of lymphoma and three cases of NMSC in psoriasis patients with secukinumab treatment (n = 3430) [56]. Similarly, long-term pooled data from one phase II and three phase III clinical trials found 56 cases of NMSC and one case of lymphoma after receiving brodalumab (n = 4464) [57]. Moreover, data pooled from seven ixekizumab clinical trials (n = 4209) for psoriasis reported 27 cases of NMSC and two cases of lymphoma [58].

Two phase III clinical trials (Voyage 1 [n = 329] evaluated through week 48 and Voyage 2 [n = 496] evaluated through 1 year) compared the safety and efficacy of guselkumab to adalimumab in the treatment of moderate-to-severe psoriasis [59, 60]. The trials reported three cases of lymphoma and zero cases of NMSC [59, 60]. Two tildrakizumab phase III clinical trials (n = 1238) also reported low rates of NMSC (20 cases) and lymphoma (zero cases) through week 148 in patients with moderate-to-severe psoriasis [61]. Risankizumab is another IL-23 inhibitor with low reported cases of NMSC (incidence ratio 0.3) and lymphoma (0 cases) [62, 63].

The risk of malignancy with TNF-alpha inhibitor therapy in psoriasis patients has been well reported in the literature due to the suppression of inflammatory pathways related to cancer development [64, 65]. Moreover, the FDA has issued a black-box warning for the risk of non-Hodgkin lymphoma in patients treated with TNF inhibitors [66]. A retrospective cohort study of rheumatologic conditions, including psoriatic arthritis, supported the FDA warning reporting a significant risk of non-Hodgkin lymphoma with any exposure to TNF inhibitors (odds ratio (OR) = 1.93; 95% confidence interval (CI): 1.16–3.20) [67]. However, a recent meta-analysis of TNF-alpha inhibitors in psoriasis disease reported a nonsignificant risk of NMSC (OR = 1.33; 95% CI: 0.58–3.04) [68]. Similarly, a population-based cohort study of various conditions including psoriasis reported no association between TNF-alpha inhibitor therapy and increased risk of malignancy [69].

Ustekinumab is first line for patients with a history of NMSC and lymphoma with demonstrated safety and efficacy in long-term studies. Interleukin-17 inhibitors and IL-23 have a low risk of NMSC and lymphoma development. A black-box warning for lymphoma has been issued for TNF-alpha inhibitors; thus, this class is last line.

Expert opinion algorithm:

1. Ustekinumab
2. IL-17 inhibitors or IL-23 inhibitors
3. TNF-alpha inhibitors (avoid in lymphoma).

Biologics for Geriatric Patients

Geriatric (aged 65 or older) patients pose therapeutic complexity due to comorbid conditions and polypharmacy, which may impact the safety and efficacy of treatment with biologics [70] along with other systemic nonbiologic treatments. Data for this group are limited as geriatric patients are often excluded from clinical trials [71]. However, the National Psoriasis Foundation (NPF) recommends biologics as one of the first-line treatment agents for moderate-to-severe psoriasis in the elderly [72]. A recent meta-analysis reported an increased risk of infection in elderly patients (>60 years old, n = 4719) receiving biologic therapy for chronic immune conditions including psoriasis compared to elderly patients not receiving biologic therapy (n = 3961) and younger patients (n = 13,305) receiving biologic therapy, with a pooled OR of 2.28 (95% CI: 1.57–3.31) [73]. However, the elderly patients on biologics did not show an increased risk of malignancy (OR = 0.54, 95% CI: 0.28–1.05) or mortality (OR = 1.52, 95% CI: 0.44–5.20) compared to nonbiologic elderly patients [73]. While vaccination has not been shown to reduce infection rates, patients should receive necessary recommended vaccines before initiation of biologics, with only killed vaccines being provided during treatment with biologics [72]. Additionally, special attention is needed when evaluating geriatric patients for psoriatic plaques in intertriginous areas, such as the intergluteal folds and axillae [72].

As of July 14, 2021, no studies of IL-23 inhibitors in the elderly are available on PubMed. The FDA drug-prescribing information for risankizumab reported comparable safety and efficacy between younger and geriatric patients ages ≥65 (n = 243) and ≥75 (n = 24). However, caution is advised as the report states the number of subjects was not sufficient to determine a variance in treatment response between the two groups [24]. Similarly, the FDA-prescribing information for tildrakizumab reported similar findings for 92 patients aged 65 or older and 17 patients aged 75 or older with exposure to the biologic [25]. Guselkumab also reports similar data for 93 patients aged 65 or older and four patients aged 75 or older [23].

Ustekinumab has demonstrated low rates of infection in this population. A retrospective study of 24 psoriasis patients showed 60% of patients achieving PASI 75 at week 52, with none of the patients developing severe infections after 1 year [74]. Higher efficacy was demonstrated in a study of 22 elderly patients with psoriasis after 90.9% of patients achieved PASI 75 by 100 weeks, without any infections in the following 2 years [75].

In a multicenter retrospective cohort study of psoriasis patients treated with secukinumab (n = 72), ixekizumab (n = 35), and brodalumab (n = 7), 80 patients (70%) achieved Physician

Global Assessment and Body Surface Area (PGA) score of 0/1 after 6 months [76]. Of note, some patients had to discontinue treatment due to multiple reasons including primary treatment failure (n = 11), disease relapse (n = 14), or adverse events (n = 7, e.g., injection site reactions, oral candidiasis, and influenza-like illnesses) [76]. A pooled analysis of three phase III randomized clinical trials compared elderly patients (aged ≥65 years, n = 67) to younger patients (aged 18–64, n = 841) with moderate-to-severe psoriasis [77]. The study demonstrated PASI 75 is achieved by a higher number of geriatric patients (81.8%) compared to younger patients (79.4%) at 52 weeks, with similar rates of adverse events for the two groups [77]. Also, a post hoc analysis of 67 elderly psoriasis patients (≥65 years) treated with secukinumab reported treatment safety and efficacy being comparable to younger patients (PASI 75 at 52 weeks: elderly 81.8%, younger 79.4%), even with a greater prevalence of comorbid cardiovascular and metabolic conditions in the elderly group [77]. In another two-year retrospective study of geriatric (aged ≥ 65) psoriasis patients (n = 29) treated with secukinumab and other concomitant medications, six patients had to discontinue treatment [78]. Five of the patients discontinued treatment due to lack of efficacy, while the last patient discontinued secukinumab treatment due to fevers and tremors that completely resolved following secukinumab treatment cessation. The remaining patients were reported to have a PASI score (mean ± SD) of 1.7 ± 1.9 ($p < 0.001$) starting from a baseline of 11.4 ± 6.3, with a mean PASI reduction of 85.1% [78]. A case report also reported similar findings in an 85-year-old female with comorbid conditions and polypharmacy [79]. The FDA-prescribing information for ixekizumab reported no differences in safety and efficacy for 301 patients (aged ≥ 65) and 36 patients (aged ≥ 75) compared to younger patients in a total of 4204 psoriasis subjects with ixekizumab exposure while also stating the sample might not be sufficient to observe differences in treatment response [22]. A different retrospective cohort study of 16 elderly psoriasis patients reported PASI 100 of 81.2% at week 48 for 15 of the patients, as one discontinued due to psoriatic arthritic symptoms [80].

Tumor necrosis factor inhibitors should be used with caution in elderly psoriasis patients due to the potential for an increased risk of adverse events. Psoriasis is a well-established risk factor for cardiovascular disease and new-onset congestive heart failure, conditions that have an increased prevalence in the elderly, and can be exacerbated by TNF-alpha inhibitors [81–85]. Additionally, TNF-alpha inhibitors have a black-box warning for risk of tuberculosis, among other infections, which can adversely affect the elderly who are already immunocompromised [86]. In the analysis of a phase III adalimumab clinical trial of psoriasis patients, the study reported a decreased treatment response for elderly subgroups (aged ≥ 65, n = 54) compared to younger subgroups (aged < 65) with fewer elderly patients (64%) achieving PASI 75 by week 16 compared to patients aged 40–64 (n = 318; 70%) and patients aged <40 (n = 225; 74%) [87, 88]. Similarly, in a retrospective cohort study of aged 65 and older geriatric patients with psoriasis (n = 16), the safety of the biologic treatment was demonstrated with only two patients experiencing adverse events (e.g., EBV infection and hemorrhagic cystitis) [89]. Another retrospective study of elderly (aged ≥ 65) psoriasis patients treated with adalimumab (n = 28) and etanercept (n = 61) reported adequate safety profiles for both agents with PASI 75 of 71.43% and 83.61% at 156 weeks for the adalimumab and etanercept groups, respectively [90]. In another retrospective study, infliximab demonstrated efficacy in elderly (aged 65–85) psoriasis (n = 12) and psoriatic arthritis patients (n = 14), with reduction in the mean PASI score being maintained through week 208 compared to a PASI baseline score (mean ± SD) of 15.6 ± 10.2 in 12 patients ($p < 0.001$) [91]. A multicenter retrospective study (n = 266) examined elderly psoriatic patients (aged ≥ 65) treated with adalimumab (31.2%), ustekinumab (28.9%), etanercept (20.3%), secukinumab (15%), infliximab (3%), golimumab (1%), and certolizumab pegol (0.6%) demonstrated safety and efficacy for all drugs examined [92]. After 52 weeks, a PASI score (mean ± SD) of 1.2 ± 2.1 was achieved from a baseline of 16.5 ± 7.1. Twenty-five adverse events were reported, with the majority being infections ($n = 12$) and malignancy ($n = 4$). However, the study stated the adverse event rates were comparable to younger populations [92]. Lastly, an observational study of 187 psoriasis patients older than 65 years of age reported the following percentage of patients achieving PASI 75 at 12 weeks of therapy: ustekinumab (100%), infliximab (93.3%), adalimumab (64.7%), and etanercept (64.1%) [93]. The adverse events rates per patient-year were lowest for etanercept (0.11) and highest for adalimumab (0.35) [93].

Expert opinion algorithm:

1. IL-23 inhibitors or ustekinumab
2. IL-17 inhibitors
3. TNF-alpha inhibitors.

Biologics for Patients Undergoing Surgery

Only a limited number of studies specifically evaluating the efficacy and safety of psoriasis patients undergoing surgery receiving biologic treatment have been published. A greater number of studies exploring the risks and benefits of perioperative biologic use have been conducted in patients in other autoimmune conditions, such as rheumatoid arthritis and inflammatory bowel disease [94–97]. When deciding whether to continue or withhold biologics in the perioperative period, the risk of infection and delayed wound healing should be weighed against the risk of inducing a psoriasis disease flare, among additional patient-specific factors [94, 98].

Data and studies for IL-17 inhibitors and IL-23 inhibitors are limited. A PubMed and FDA-prescribing information search performed on July 12, 2021, did not yield any results for IL-17 inhibitors and IL-23 inhibitors in psoriasis patients undergoing surgery [21–25, 99].

A large retrospective study ($n = 827$) of patients on adalimumab ($n = 66$), infliximab ($n = 68$), etanercept ($n = 49$), and ustekinumab ($n = 35$), 27.2% of who had psoriasis, found no statistically significant difference in skin and soft tissue infection rates (includes perioperative and non-perioperative time periods) across the four biologics ($p = 0.49$) [100]. However, ustekinumab was found to have the lowest rate of skin and soft tissue infections (8.2%), while etanercept was found to have the highest rate (13.7%) [100]. Although further studies conducted in patients with psoriasis are limited for this biologic class, a retrospective study compared perioperative ustekinumab ($n = 44$) to perioperative TNF inhibitor ($n = 169$) exposure in Crohn's disease patients [97]. This study reported a nonsignificant lower risk of surgery site infection in ustekinumab (13%) compared to TNF inhibitors (20%) within 30 days of surgery [97]. Ustekinumab had a higher rate of return to the operating room ($p = 0.01$), which the authors stated could be due to differences in referral center practices as one center accounted for most of the returns [97]. Another study comparing ustekinumab to vedolizumab in 103 Crohn's disease patients did not report a significant increase in perioperative complication rates after comparing 26 matched patients [101].

In 2014, a retrospective study of 131 patients with psoriasis (118 on TNF-alpha inhibitors and 13 on ustekinumab) noted no significant difference in the rate of psoriasis flares or perioperative infections in patients continuing or discontinuing biologics in the perioperative period [102]. A subsequent retrospective study of psoriasis and/or psoriatic arthritis patients ($n = 42$), predominantly treated with TNF-alpha inhibitors (89%), also showed no significant difference in the rate of perioperative infections or delayed wound healing between patients continuing biologics and patients discontinuing biologics [103]. Notably, interruption of biologic use during the perioperative period was associated with a significant risk ($p = 0.003$) of psoriasis or psoriatic arthritis disease flare [103]. Similarly, a subsequent retrospective study of psoriasis patients (n = 48), predominately on TNF-alpha inhibitors (85%), demonstrated no evidence of higher complication rates associated with perioperative biologic use [104]. Moreover, a small retrospective study of 19 elective surgeries (6 major and 13 minor surgeries) performed in 17 psoriasis patients on TNF-alpha inhibitors reported surgical site infection development in two patients continuing etanercept perioperatively and psoriasis flare in 5/6 patients discontinuing anti-TNF-alpha agents perioperatively [105]. Lastly, a case series of four psoriasis patients undergoing surgery with TNF-alpha inhibitor exposure reported zero surgical complications in three patients, while one patient had a recurrence of psoriasis, which subsequently improved after biologic re-initiation [106].

The 2019 Joint American Academy of Dermatology-NPF guidelines of care for the management and treatment of psoriasis recommends all biologics be continued perioperatively for low-risk procedures [30]. However, moderate- and high-risk procedures should be approached on a case-by-case basis in collaboration with the surgical team. If discontinuation of the biologic is deemed necessary, the biologic should be withheld for 3–4 half-lives before, and 1–2 weeks after, surgery in the absence of complications [30]. Similar recommendations were made in a 2016 review from the Medical Board of the NPF [107].

Overall, IL-17 inhibitors and IL-23 inhibitors do not have published studies for psoriasis patients undergoing surgery. For all other classes of approved biologics for the treatment of psoriasis, it is imperative to weigh the risks of infection and delayed wound healing (procedure and patient-dependent) against the risk inducing a psoriasis flare (patient-dependent) when deciding if and when to withhold biologics perioperatively [94].

Expert opinion algorithm:

4. IL-23 inhibitors or ustekinumab
5. IL-17 inhibitors
6. TNF-alpha inhibitors.

Role of Biomarkers/Precision Medicine with Psoriasis Biologics

Recent recommendations from the NPF call for biomarkers and precision medicine use when treating psoriasis patients with biologics to help identify optimal therapeutics that could reduce disease onset and disease burden. Targeted therapies could help alleviate the financial/medical burden and reduce discontinuation of treatment or biologic class switching due to lack of treatment response [30, 108, 109]. One option is Mind.Px, an emerging analytical predictive tool combining skin data, biomarkers, and artificial intelligence/machine learning through collaboration by multiple industry sectors [110]. This tool is stated to help guide physicians in selecting the optimal biologic therapies based on individual patient genetic markers. By analyzing over 7000 biomarkers in RNA samples collected from a patient's psoriasis plaque, the tool predicts responsiveness to a biologic class with the goal of improving clinical outcomes and reducing associated costs [110].

Conclusion

Improved understanding of the pathogenesis of psoriasis and increased recognition of comorbid conditions have led to an increase in available FDA-approved therapeutic options. The development of numerous classes of biologics offers patients and clinicians flexibility in selecting the optimal treatment choice. This chapter aims to serve as a guide for healthcare providers in selecting a biologic agent by providing treatment algorithms for special populations including, pregnancy and breastfeeding, HIV, history of NMSC, history of lymphoma, geriatric patients, and patients undergoing surgery (Table 11.1). Additionally, this chapter highlights an upcoming precision medicine tool, which uses biomarkers to guide biologic choice in psoriasis clinical management. As further trials report on long-term safety and efficacy data with the approval of new classes of biologics, treatment recommendations need to be altered accordingly.

Table 11.1 Our evidence-based biologic treatment algorithms for special populations

	Pregnancy and breastfeeding	HIV-positive	History of NMSC and lymphoma	Geriatric patients	Undergoing surgery
TNF-alpha inhibitors					
Adalimumab	Fourth line	First line[a]	Third line (avoid in lymphoma)	Third line	Third line
Etanercept	Second line	First line[a]	Third line (avoid in lymphoma)	Third line	Third line
Infliximab	Fourth line	First line[a]	Third line (avoid in lymphoma)	Third line	Third line
Certolizumab pegol	First line	First line[a]	Third line (avoid in lymphoma)	Third line	Third line
IL-12/23 inhibitors					
Ustekinumab	Third line[b]	First line[a]	First line	First line	First line
IL-17 inhibitors					
Ixekizumab	Fifth line	Second line	Second line	Second line	Second line
Secukinumab	Third line[b]	Second line	Second line	Second line	Second line
Brodalumab	Fifth line	Second line	Second line	Second line	Second line
IL-23p19 inhibitors					
Guselkumab	Fifth line	Second line	Second line	First line	First line
Tildrakizumab	Fifth line	Second line	Second line	First line	First line
Risankizumab	Fifth line	Second line	Second line	First line	First line

IL interleukin, *TNF* tumor necrosis factor, *HIV* human immunodeficiency virus, *NMSC* nonmelanoma skin cancer
[a]Patients must be receiving highly active retroviral therapy, have a normal CD4+ count, and have no recent history of opportunistic infections
[b]Class B drug with old pregnancy classes

References

1. Rich SJ, Bello-Quintero CE. Advancements in the treatment of psoriasis: role of biologic agents. J Manag Care Pharm. 2004;10(4):318–25. https://doi.org/10.18553/jmcp.2004.10.4.318.
2. Brownstone ND, Hong J, Mosca M, Hadeler E, Liao W, Bhutani T, et al. Biologic treatments of psoriasis: an update for the clinician. Biologics. 2021;15:39–51. https://doi.org/10.2147/BTT.S252578.
3. Strober B, Karki C, Mason M, Guo N, Holmgren SH, Greenberg JD, et al. Characterization of disease burden, comorbidities, and treatment use in a large, US-based cohort: results from the Corrona Psoriasis Registry. J Am Acad Dermatol. 2018;78(2):323–32. https://doi.org/10.1016/j.jaad.2017.10.012.
4. Amin M, No DJ, Egeberg A, Wu JJ. Choosing first-line biologic treatment for moderate-to-severe psoriasis: what does the evidence say? Am J Clin Dermatol. 2018;19(1):1–13. https://doi.org/10.1007/s40257-017-0328-3.
5. Galluzzo M, D'Adamio S, Bianchi L, Talamonti M. Psoriasis in pregnancy: case series and literature review of data concerning exposure during pregnancy to ustekinumab. J Dermatolog Treat. 2019;30(1):40–4. https://doi.org/10.1080/09546634.2018.1468066.
6. Ferreira C, Azevedo A, Nogueira M, Torres T. Management of psoriasis in pregnancy - a review of the evidence to date. Drugs Context. 2020;9. https://doi.org/10.7573/dic.2019-11-6.
7. Mariette X, Förger F, Abraham B, Flynn AD, Moltó A, Flipo RM, et al. Lack of placental transfer of certolizumab pegol during pregnancy: results from CRIB, a prospective, postmarketing, pharmacokinetic study. Ann Rheum Dis. 2018;77(2):228–33. https://doi.org/10.1136/annrheumdis-2017-212196.
8. Clowse MEB, Scheuerle AE, Chambers C, Afzali A, Kimball AB, Cush JJ, et al. Pregnancy outcomes

after exposure to certolizumab pegol: updated results from a pharmacovigilance safety database. Arthritis Rheumatol. 2018;70(9):1399–407. https://doi.org/10.1002/art.40508.
9. Clowse ME, Förger F, Hwang C, Thorp J, Dolhain RJ, van Tubergen A, et al. Minimal to no transfer of certolizumab pegol into breast milk: results from CRADLE, a prospective, postmarketing, multicentre, pharmacokinetic study. Ann Rheum Dis. 2017;76(11):1890–6. https://doi.org/10.1136/annrheumdis-2017-211384.
10. Porter ML, Lockwood SJ, Kimball AB. Update on biologic safety for patients with psoriasis during pregnancy. Int J Womens Dermatol. 2017;3(1):21–5. https://doi.org/10.1016/j.ijwd.2016.12.003.
11. Eworuke E, Panucci G, Goulding M, Neuner R, Toh S. Use of tumor necrosis factor-alpha inhibitors during pregnancy among women who delivered live born infants. Pharmacoepidemiol Drug Saf. 2019;28(3):296–304. https://doi.org/10.1002/pds.4695.
12. Bröms G, Kieler H, Ekbom A, Gissler M, Hellgren K, Lahesmaa-Korpinen AM, et al. Anti-TNF treatment during pregnancy and birth outcomes: a population-based study from Denmark, Finland, and Sweden. Pharmacoepidemiol Drug Saf. 2020;29(3):316–27. https://doi.org/10.1002/pds.4930.
13. Lund T, Thomsen SF. Use of TNF-inhibitors and ustekinumab for psoriasis during pregnancy: a patient series. Dermatol Ther. 2017;30(3). https://doi.org/10.1111/dth.12454.
14. Watson N, Wu K, Farr P, Reynolds NJ, Hampton PJ. Ustekinumab exposure during conception and pregnancy in patients with chronic plaque psoriasis: a case series of 10 pregnancies. Br J Dermatol. 2019;180(1):195–6. https://doi.org/10.1111/bjd.17086.
15. Andrulonis R, Ferris LK. Treatment of severe psoriasis with ustekinumab during pregnancy. J Drugs Dermatol. 2012;11(10):1240.
16. Rocha K, Piccinin MC, Kalache LF, Reichert-Faria A, Silva de Castro CC. Pregnancy during ustekinumab treatment for severe psoriasis. Dermatology. 2015;231(2):103–4. https://doi.org/10.1159/000380880.
17. Alsenaid A, Prinz JC. Inadvertent pregnancy during ustekinumab therapy in a patient with plaque psoriasis and impetigo herpetiformis. J Eur Acad Dermatol Venereol. 2016;30(3):488–90. https://doi.org/10.1111/jdv.12872.
18. Sheeran C, Nicolopoulos J. Pregnancy outcomes of two patients exposed to ustekinumab in the first trimester. Australas J Dermatol. 2014;55(3):235–6. https://doi.org/10.1111/ajd.12214.
19. MotherToBaby: Ustekinumab (Stelara®) Fact Sheet. https://mothertobaby.org/fact-sheets/ustekinumab-pregnancy/pdf/ (2019). Accessed 27 Nov 2020.
20. Warren RB, Reich K, Langley RG, Strober B, Gladman D, Deodhar A, et al. Secukinumab in pregnancy: outcomes in psoriasis, psoriatic arthritis and ankylosing spondylitis from the global safety database. Br J Dermatol. 2018;179(5):1205–7. https://doi.org/10.1111/bjd.16901.
21. AstraZeneca I: SILIQTM (brodalumab) injection, for subcutaneous use. https://www.accessdata.fda.gov/drugsatfda_docs/label/2017/761032lbl.pdf (2017). Accessed 12 July 2021.
22. Company ELa: TALTZ (ixekizumab) injection, for subcutaneous use: US prescribing information. https://www.accessdata.fda.gov/drugsatfda_docs/label/2017/125521s004lbl.pdf (2016). Accessed 12 July 2021.
23. Janssen Biotech I: Tremfya™ (guselkumab) injection, for subcutaneous use: US prescribing information. https://www.accessdata.fda.gov/drugsatfda_docs/label/2017/761061s000lbl.pdf (2017). Accessed 12 July 2021.
24. Abbvie I: SKYRIZITM (risankizumab-rzaa) injection, for subcutaneous use: US prescribing information. https://www.accessdata.fda.gov/drugsatfda_docs/label/2019/761105s000lbl.pdf (2019). Accessed 12 July 2021.
25. Sun Pharma I: ILUMYATM (tildrakizumab-asmn) injection, for subcutaneous use: US prescribing information. https://www.accessdata.fda.gov/drugsatfda_docs/label/2018/761067s000lbl.pdf#page=10 (2018). Accessed 12 July 2021.
26. Prevention CfDCa: HIV Basics. https://www.cdc.gov/hiv/basics/statistics.html (2021). Accessed 30 June 2021.
27. Menon K, Van Voorhees AS, Bebo BF Jr, Gladman DD, Hsu S, Kalb RE, et al. Psoriasis in patients with HIV infection: from the medical board of the National Psoriasis Foundation. J Am Acad Dermatol. 2010;62(2):291–9. https://doi.org/10.1016/j.jaad.2009.03.047.
28. Fife DJ, Waller JM, Jeffes EW, Koo JY. Unraveling the paradoxes of HIV-associated psoriasis: a review of T-cell subsets and cytokine profiles. Dermatol Online J. 2007;13(2):4.
29. Armstrong AW: Treatment selection for moderate to severe plaque psoriasis in special populations. https://www.uptodate.com/contents/treatment-selection-for-moderate-to-severe-plaque-psoriasis-in-special-populations#H9475354 (2020). Accessed 14 July 2021.
30. Menter A, Strober BE, Kaplan DH, Kivelevitch D, Prater EF, Stoff B, et al. Joint AAD-NPF guidelines of care for the management and treatment of psoriasis with biologics. J Am Acad Dermatol. 2019;80(4):1029–72. https://doi.org/10.1016/j.jaad.2018.11.057.
31. Nicoletta B, Alessandra N, Nevena S, Tolino E, Colapietra D, Claudio M, et al. Management of psoriatic patients in biologic treatment associated with infectious comorbidities. Postepy Dermatol Alergol. 2020;37(3):417–21. https://doi.org/10.5114/ada.2020.96155.
32. Aboulafia DM, Bundow D, Wilske K, Ochs UI. Etanercept for the treatment of human

immunodeficiency virus-associated psoriatic arthritis. Mayo Clin Proc. 2000;75(10):1093–8. https://doi.org/10.4065/75.10.1093.
33. Lee ES, Heller MM, Kamangar F, Park KK, Koo JY. Long-term etanercept use for severe generalized psoriasis in an HIV-infected individual: a case study. J Drugs Dermatol. 2012;11(3):413–4.
34. Mikhail M, Weinberg JM, Smith BL. Successful treatment with etanercept of von Zumbusch pustular psoriasis in a patient with human immunodeficiency virus. Arch Dermatol. 2008;144(4):453–6. https://doi.org/10.1001/archderm.144.4.453.
35. De Simone C, Perino F, Caldarola G, D'Agostino M, Peris K. Treatment of psoriasis with etanercept in immunocompromised patients: two case reports. J Int Med Res. 2016;44(1 suppl):67–71. https://doi.org/10.1177/0300060515593250.
36. Paparizos V, Rallis E, Kirsten L, Kyriakis K. Ustekinumab for the treatment of HIV psoriasis. J Dermatolog Treat. 2012;23(6):398–9. https://doi.org/10.3109/09546634.2011.579085.
37. Saeki H, Ito T, Hayashi M, Fukuchi O, Umezawa Y, Nobeyama Y, et al. Successful treatment of ustekinumab in a severe psoriasis patient with human immunodeficiency virus infection. J Eur Acad Dermatol Venereol. 2015;29(8):1653–5. https://doi.org/10.1111/jdv.12531.
38. Lindsey SF, Weiss J, Lee ES, Romanelli P. Treatment of severe psoriasis and psoriatic arthritis with adalimumab in an HIV-positive patient. J Drugs Dermatol. 2014;13(7):869–71.
39. Montes-Torres A, Aparicio G, Rivera R, Vilarrasa E, Marcellán M, Notario J, et al. Safety and effectiveness of conventional systemic therapy and biological drugs in patients with moderate to severe psoriasis and HIV infection: a retrospective multicenter study. J Dermatolog Treat. 2019;30(5):461–5. https://doi.org/10.1080/09546634.2018.1535690.
40. Bardazzi F, Magnano M, Campanati A, Loconsole F, Carpentieri A, Potenza C, et al. Biologic therapies in HIV-infected patients with psoriasis: an Italian experience. Acta Derm Venereol. 2017;97(8):989–90. https://doi.org/10.2340/00015555-2698.
41. UCB I: CIMZIA (certolizumab pegol) for injection, for subcutaneous use: US prescribing information. https://www.accessdata.fda.gov/drugsatfda_docs/label/2017/125160s270lbl.pdf (2017). Accessed 12 July 2021.
42. Pangilinan MCG, Sermswan P, Asawanonda P. Use of anti-IL-17 monoclonal antibodies in HIV patients with erythrodermic psoriasis. Case Rep Dermatol. 2020;12(2):132–7. https://doi.org/10.1159/000508781.
43. Di Lernia V, Casanova DM, Garlassi E. Secukinumab in an HIV-positive patient with psoriasis. J Dtsch Dermatol Ges. 2019;17(6):646–8. https://doi.org/10.1111/ddg.13851.
44. Pouplard C, Brenaut E, Horreau C, Barnetche T, Misery L, Richard MA, et al. Risk of cancer in psoriasis: a systematic review and meta-analysis of epidemiological studies. J Eur Acad Dermatol Venereol. 2013;27 Suppl 3:36–46. https://doi.org/10.1111/jdv.12165.
45. Lee MS, Lin RY, Chang YT, Lai MS. The risk of developing non-melanoma skin cancer, lymphoma and melanoma in patients with psoriasis in Taiwan: a 10-year, population-based cohort study. Int J Dermatol. 2012;51(12):1454–60. https://doi.org/10.1111/j.1365-4632.2011.05310.x.
46. Takeshita J, Grewal S, Langan SM, Mehta NN, Ogdie A, Van Voorhees AS, et al. Psoriasis and comorbid diseases: epidemiology. J Am Acad Dermatol. 2017;76(3):377–90. https://doi.org/10.1016/j.jaad.2016.07.064.
47. Gelfand JM, Shin DB, Neimann AL, Wang X, Margolis DJ, Troxel AB. The risk of lymphoma in patients with psoriasis. J Invest Dermatol. 2006;126(10):2194–201. https://doi.org/10.1038/sj.jid.5700410.
48. Chiesa Fuxench ZC, Shin DB, Ogdie Beatty A, Gelfand JM. The risk of cancer in patients with psoriasis: a population-based cohort study in the health improvement network. JAMA Dermatol. 2016;152(3):282–90. https://doi.org/10.1001/jamadermatol.2015.4847.
49. Lebwohl M, Leonardi C, Griffiths CE, Prinz JC, Szapary PO, Yeilding N, et al. Long-term safety experience of ustekinumab in patients with moderate-to-severe psoriasis (part I of II): results from analyses of general safety parameters from pooled phase 2 and 3 clinical trials. J Am Acad Dermatol. 2012;66(5):731–41. https://doi.org/10.1016/j.jaad.2011.06.011.
50. Gordon KB, Papp KA, Langley RG, Ho V, Kimball AB, Guzzo C, et al. Long-term safety experience of ustekinumab in patients with moderate to severe psoriasis (part II of II): results from analyses of infections and malignancy from pooled phase II and III clinical trials. J Am Acad Dermatol. 2012;66(5):742–51. https://doi.org/10.1016/j.jaad.2011.06.041.
51. Papp KA, Griffiths CE, Gordon K, Lebwohl M, Szapary PO, Wasfi Y, et al. Long-term safety of ustekinumab in patients with moderate-to-severe psoriasis: final results from 5 years of follow-up. Br J Dermatol. 2013;168(4):844–54. https://doi.org/10.1111/bjd.12214.
52. Charakopoulos E, Spyrou I, Viniou NA, Giannakopoulou N, Hatzidavid S, Diamantopoulos PT. A case report of Hodgkin lymphoma in a patient treated with ustekinumab for psoriasis. Medicine (Baltimore). 2020;99(21):e20048. https://doi.org/10.1097/md.0000000000020048.
53. Lasek W, Zagożdżon R, Jakobisiak M. Interleukin 12: still a promising candidate for tumor immunotherapy? Cancer Immunol Immunother. 2014;63(5):419–35. https://doi.org/10.1007/s00262-014-1523-1.
54. Papp K, Gottlieb AB, Naldi L, Pariser D, Ho V, Goyal K, et al. Safety surveillance for ustekinumab and other psoriasis treatments from the psoriasis

longitudinal assessment and registry (PSOLAR). J Drugs Dermatol. 2015;14(7):706–14.
55. Zou W, Restifo NP. T(H)17 cells in tumour immunity and immunotherapy. Nat Rev Immunol. 2010;10(4):248–56. https://doi.org/10.1038/nri2742.
56. van de Kerkhof PC, Griffiths CE, Reich K, Leonardi CL, Blauvelt A, Tsai TF, et al. Secukinumab long-term safety experience: a pooled analysis of 10 phase II and III clinical studies in patients with moderate to severe plaque psoriasis. J Am Acad Dermatol. 2016;75(1):83–98.e4. https://doi.org/10.1016/j.jaad.2016.03.024.
57. Gottlieb A, Lebwohl M, Liu C, Israel RJ, Jacobson A. Malignancy rates in brodalumab clinical studies for psoriasis. Am J Clin Dermatol. 2020;21(3):421–30. https://doi.org/10.1007/s40257-020-00512-4.
58. Strober B, Leonardi C, Papp KA, Mrowietz U, Ohtsuki M, Bissonnette R, et al. Short- and long-term safety outcomes with ixekizumab from 7 clinical trials in psoriasis: Etanercept comparisons and integrated data. J Am Acad Dermatol. 2017;76(3):432–40.e17. https://doi.org/10.1016/j.jaad.2016.09.026.
59. Blauvelt A, Papp KA, Griffiths CE, Randazzo B, Wasfi Y, Shen YK, et al. Efficacy and safety of guselkumab, an anti-interleukin-23 monoclonal antibody, compared with adalimumab for the continuous treatment of patients with moderate to severe psoriasis: results from the phase III, double-blinded, placebo- and active comparator-controlled VOYAGE 1 trial. J Am Acad Dermatol. 2017;76(3):405–17. https://doi.org/10.1016/j.jaad.2016.11.041.
60. Reich K, Armstrong AW, Foley P, Song M, Wasfi Y, Randazzo B, et al. Efficacy and safety of guselkumab, an anti-interleukin-23 monoclonal antibody, compared with adalimumab for the treatment of patients with moderate to severe psoriasis with randomized withdrawal and retreatment: results from the phase III, double-blind, placebo- and active comparator-controlled VOYAGE 2 trial. J Am Acad Dermatol. 2017;76(3):418–31. https://doi.org/10.1016/j.jaad.2016.11.042.
61. Reich K, Warren RB, Iversen L, Puig L, Pau-Charles I, Igarashi A, et al. Long-term efficacy and safety of tildrakizumab for moderate-to-severe psoriasis: pooled analyses of two randomized phase III clinical trials (reSURFACE 1 and reSURFACE 2) through 148 weeks. Br J Dermatol. 2020;182(3):605–17. https://doi.org/10.1111/bjd.18232.
62. Gordon KB, Strober B, Lebwohl M, Augustin M, Blauvelt A, Poulin Y, et al. Efficacy and safety of risankizumab in moderate-to-severe plaque psoriasis (UltIMMa-1 and UltIMMa-2): results from two double-blind, randomised, placebo-controlled and ustekinumab-controlled phase 3 trials. Lancet. 2018;392(10148):650–61. https://doi.org/10.1016/s0140-6736(18)31713-6.
63. Bachelez H, Gordon K, Blauvelt A, Wu J, Sinvhal R, Photowala H, et al. Short- and long-term safety of risankizumab in patients with moderate to-severe psoriasis: an integrated analysis. J Eur Acad Dermatol Venereol. 2019;33:37–8. ISBN/ISSN: 09269959
64. Peleva E, Exton LS, Kelley K, Kleyn CE, Mason KJ, Smith CH. Risk of cancer in patients with psoriasis on biological therapies: a systematic review. Br J Dermatol. 2018;178(1):103–13. https://doi.org/10.1111/bjd.15830.
65. van Lümig PP, Menting SP, van den Reek JM, Spuls PI, van Riel PL, van de Kerkhof PC, et al. An increased risk of non-melanoma skin cancer during TNF-inhibitor treatment in psoriasis patients compared to rheumatoid arthritis patients probably relates to disease-related factors. J Eur Acad Dermatol Venereol. 2015;29(4):752–60. https://doi.org/10.1111/jdv.12675.
66. Food, Administration D. Follow-up to the June 4 2008 early communication about the ongoing safety review of tumor necrosis factor (TNF) blockers (marketed as Remicade, Enbrel, Humira, Cimzia, and Simponi).
67. Calip GS, Patel PR, Adimadhyam S, Xing S, Wu Z, Sweiss K, et al. Tumor necrosis factor-alpha inhibitors and risk of non-Hodgkin lymphoma in a cohort of adults with rheumatologic conditions. Int J Cancer. 2018;143(5):1062–71. https://doi.org/10.1002/ijc.31407.
68. Dommasch ED, Abuabara K, Shin DB, Nguyen J, Troxel AB, Gelfand JM. The risk of infection and malignancy with tumor necrosis factor antagonists in adults with psoriatic disease: a systematic review and meta-analysis of randomized controlled trials. J Am Acad Dermatol. 2011;64(6):1035–50. https://doi.org/10.1016/j.jaad.2010.09.734.
69. Waljee AK, Higgins PDR, Jensen CB, Villumsen M, Cohen-Mekelburg SA, Wallace BI, et al. Anti-tumour necrosis factor-α therapy and recurrent or new primary cancers in patients with inflammatory bowel disease, rheumatoid arthritis, or psoriasis and previous cancer in Denmark: a nationwide, population-based cohort study. Lancet Gastroenterol Hepatol. 2020;5(3):276–84. https://doi.org/10.1016/s2468-1253(19)30362-0.
70. Phan C, Sigal ML, Estève E, Reguiai Z, Barthélémy H, Beneton N, et al. Psoriasis in the elderly: epidemiological and clinical aspects, and evaluation of patients with very late onset psoriasis. J Eur Acad Dermatol Venereol. 2016;30(1):78–82. https://doi.org/10.1111/jdv.12850.
71. Di Lernia V, Goldust M. An overview of the efficacy and safety of systemic treatments for psoriasis in the elderly. Expert Opin Biol Ther. 2018;18(8):897–903. https://doi.org/10.1080/14712598.2018.1504016.
72. Grozdev IS, Van Voorhees AS, Gottlieb AB, Hsu S, Lebwohl MG, Bebo BF Jr, et al. Psoriasis in the elderly: from the Medical Board of the National Psoriasis Foundation. J Am Acad Dermatol. 2011;65(3):537–45. https://doi.org/10.1016/j.jaad.2010.05.014.
73. Borren NZ, Ananthakrishnan AN. Safety of biologic therapy in older patients with immune-mediated

diseases: a systematic review and meta-analysis. Clin Gastroenterol Hepatol. 2019;17(9):1736–43. e4. https://doi.org/10.1016/j.cgh.2018.12.032.
74. Hayashi M, Umezawa Y, Fukuchi O, Ito T, Saeki H, Nakagawa H. Efficacy and safety of ustekinumab treatment in elderly patients with psoriasis. J Dermatol. 2014;41(11):974–80. https://doi.org/10.1111/1346-8138.12653.
75. Megna M, Napolitano M, Balato N, Monfrecola G, Villani A, Ayala F, et al. Efficacy and safety of ustekinumab in a group of 22 elderly patients with psoriasis over a 2-year period. Clin Exp Dermatol. 2016;41(5):564–6. https://doi.org/10.1111/ced.12850.
76. Phan C, Beneton N, Delaunay J, Reguiai Z, Boulard C, Fougerousse AC, et al. Effectiveness and safety of anti-interleukin-17 therapies in elderly patients with psoriasis. Acta Derm Venereol. 2020;100(18):adv00316. https://doi.org/10.2340/00015555-3678.
77. Körber A, Papavassilis C, Bhosekar V, Reinhardt M. Efficacy and safety of secukinumab in elderly subjects with moderate to severe plaque psoriasis: a pooled analysis of phase III studies. Drugs Aging. 2018;35(2):135–44. https://doi.org/10.1007/s40266-018-0520-z.
78. Megna M, Camela E, Cinelli E, Fabbrocini G. Real-life efficacy and safety of secukinumab in elderly patients with psoriasis over a 2-year period. Clin Exp Dermatol. 2020;45(7):848–52. https://doi.org/10.1111/ced.14258.
79. Ricceri F, Pescitelli L, Lazzeri L, Di Cesare A, Prignano F. First case of secukinumab successful therapy in a very elderly psoriatic patient. Dermatol Ther. 2018;31(5):e12668. https://doi.org/10.1111/dth.12668.
80. Megna M, Cinelli E, Balato A, Gallo L, Fabbrocini G. Efficacy and safety of ixekizumab in a group of 16 elderly patients with psoriasis over a 1-year period. J Eur Acad Dermatol Venereol. 2020;34(3):e152–e3. https://doi.org/10.1111/jdv.16063.
81. Khalid U, Ahlehoff O, Gislason GH, Kristensen SL, Skov L, Torp-Pedersen C, et al. Psoriasis and risk of heart failure: a nationwide cohort study. Eur J Heart Fail. 2014;16(7):743–8. https://doi.org/10.1002/ejhf.113.
82. Hugh J, Van Voorhees AS, Nijhawan RI, Bagel J, Lebwohl M, Blauvelt A, et al. From the Medical Board of the National Psoriasis Foundation: the risk of cardiovascular disease in individuals with psoriasis and the potential impact of current therapies. J Am Acad Dermatol. 2014;70(1):168–77. https://doi.org/10.1016/j.jaad.2013.09.020.
83. Caiazzo G, Fabbrocini G, Di Caprio R, Raimondo A, Scala E, Balato N, et al. Psoriasis, cardiovascular events, and biologics: lights and shadows. Front Immunol. 2018;9:1668. https://doi.org/10.3389/fimmu.2018.01668.
84. Boyer JF, Jamard B, El Mahou S, Laroche M, Mazières B, Cantagrel A, et al. New-onset acute heart failure and ventricular tachycardia after therapy with a tumor necrosis factor antagonist. Clin Exp Rheumatol. 2005;23(2):274–5.
85. Puig L. Cardiovascular risk and psoriasis: the role of biologic therapy. Actas Dermosifiliogr. 2012;103(10):853–62. https://doi.org/10.1016/j.adengl.2012.02.004.
86. Administration FaD: FDA Drug Safety Communication: Drug labels for the Tumor Necrosis Factor-alpha (TNF alpha) blockers now include warnings about infection with Legionella and Listeria bacteria. https://www.fda.gov/drugs/drug-safety-and-availability/fda-drug-safety-communication-drug-labels-tumor-necrosis-factor-alpha-tnfa-blockers-now-include (2011). Accessed 1 July 2021.
87. Menter A, Gordon KB, Leonardi CL, Gu Y, Goldblum OM. Efficacy and safety of adalimumab across subgroups of patients with moderate to severe psoriasis. J Am Acad Dermatol. 2010;63(3):448–56. https://doi.org/10.1016/j.jaad.2009.09.040.
88. Sandhu VK, Ighani A, Fleming P, Lynde CW. Biologic treatment in elderly patients with psoriasis: a systematic review. J Cutan Med Surg. 2020;24(2):174–86. https://doi.org/10.1177/1203475419897578.
89. Chiricozzi A, Zangrilli A, Bavetta M, Bianchi L, Chimenti S, Saraceno R. Real-life 9-year experience with adalimumab in psoriasis and psoriatic arthritis: results of a single-centre, retrospective study. J Eur Acad Dermatol Venereol. 2017;31(2):304–11. https://doi.org/10.1111/jdv.13771.
90. Esposito M, Giunta A, Mazzotta A, Zangrilli A, Babino G, Bavetta M, et al. Efficacy and safety of subcutaneous anti-tumor necrosis factor-alpha agents, etanercept and adalimumab, in elderly patients affected by psoriasis and psoriatic arthritis: an observational long-term study. Dermatology. 2012;225(4):312–9. https://doi.org/10.1159/000345623.
91. Chiricozzi A, Pavlidis A, Dattola A, Bianchi L, Chimenti MS, Fida M, et al. Efficacy and safety of infliximab in psoriatic patients over the age of 65. Expert Opin Drug Saf. 2016;15(11):1459–62. https://doi.org/10.1080/14740338.2016.1226279.
92. Ricceri F, Bardazzi F, Chiricozzi A, Dapavo P, Ferrara F, Mugheddu C, et al. Elderly psoriatic patients under biological therapies: an Italian experience. J Eur Acad Dermatol Venereol. 2019;33(1):143–6. https://doi.org/10.1111/jdv.15139.
93. Piaserico S, Conti A, Lo Console F, De Simone C, Prestinari F, Mazzotta A, et al. Efficacy and safety of systemic treatments for psoriasis in elderly patients. Acta Derm Venereol. 2014;94(3):293–7. https://doi.org/10.2340/00015555-1719.
94. Plachouri KM, Georgiou S. Special aspects of biologics treatment in psoriasis: management in pregnancy, lactation, surgery, renal impairment, hepatitis and tuberculosis. J Dermatolog Treat.

2019;30(7):668–73. https://doi.org/10.1080/09546634.2018.1544413.
95. Goodman SM. Rheumatoid arthritis: perioperative management of biologics and DMARDs. Semin Arthritis Rheum. 2015;44(6):627–32. https://doi.org/10.1016/j.semarthrit.2015.01.008.
96. Argollo MC, Kotze PG, Spinelli A, Gomes TNF, Danese S. The impact of biologics in surgical outcomes in ulcerative colitis. Best Pract Res Clin Gastroenterol. 2018;32-33:79–87. https://doi.org/10.1016/j.bpg.2018.05.014.
97. Lightner AL, McKenna NP, Tse CS, Hyman N, Smith R, Ovsepyan G, et al. Postoperative outcomes in ustekinumab-treated patients undergoing abdominal operations for Crohn's disease. J Crohns Colitis. 2018;12(4):402–7. https://doi.org/10.1093/ecco-jcc/jjx163.
98. Hernandez C, Emer J, Robinson JK. Perioperative management of medications for psoriasis and psoriatic arthritis: a review for the dermasurgeon. Dermatol Surg. 2008;34(4):446–59. https://doi.org/10.1111/j.1524-4725.2007.34091.x.
99. Novartis I: COSENTYX® (secukinumab) injection, for subcutaneous use: US prescribing information. https://www.accessdata.fda.gov/drugsatfda_docs/label/2016/125504s001s002lbl.pdf (2015). Accessed 1 Oct 2020.
100. Nguyen ED, Gabel CK, Kroshinsky D. Assessing the incidence of skin and soft tissue infection in patients on biologics. J Am Acad Dermatol. 2020; https://doi.org/10.1016/j.jaad.2020.03.128.
101. Novello M, Stocchi L, Holubar S, Shawki S, Lipman J, Gorgun E, et al. Surgical outcomes of patients treated with ustekinumab vs. vedolizumab in inflammatory bowel disease: a matched case analysis. Int J Color Dis. 2019;34(3):451–7. https://doi.org/10.1007/s00384-018-3212-6.
102. Fabiano A, De Simone C, Gisondi P, Piaserico S, Lasagni C, Pellacani G, et al. Management of patients with psoriasis treated with biological drugs needing a surgical treatment. Drug Dev Res. 2014;75 Suppl 1:S24–6. https://doi.org/10.1002/ddr.21189.
103. Bakkour W, Purssell H, Chinoy H, Griffiths CE, Warren RB. The risk of post-operative complications in psoriasis and psoriatic arthritis patients on biologic therapy undergoing surgical procedures. J Eur Acad Dermatol Venereol. 2016;30(1):86–91. https://doi.org/10.1111/jdv.12997.
104. Galiano Mejías S, Carretero G, Ferrandiz C, Vanaclocha F, Daudén E, Gómez-García FJ, et al. Management of biologic therapy in moderate to severe psoriasis in surgical patients: data from the Spanish Biobadaderm registry. Actas Dermosifiliogr. 2017;108(1):52–8. https://doi.org/10.1016/j.ad.2016.08.003.
105. Reinstadler A, Mau N, Bhutani T, Talkin B, Yamauchi P, Chiu M, et al. Perioperative use of anti-tumor necrosis factor-alfa agents. J Am Acad Dermatol. 2010;62(1):154–5. https://doi.org/10.1016/j.jaad.2009.04.039.
106. Kawakami H, Matsumoto Y, Abe N, Katori Y, Takahashi K, Tsuboi R, et al. Perioperative management of tumor necrosis factor-alpha blocker-treated psoriatic patients: case reports and review. J Dermatol. 2016;43(2):190–3. https://doi.org/10.1111/1346-8138.13047.
107. Choi YM, Debbaneh M, Weinberg JM, Yamauchi PS, Van Voorhees AS, Armstrong AW, et al. From the Medical Board of the National Psoriasis Foundation: perioperative management of systemic immunomodulatory agents in patients with psoriasis and psoriatic arthritis. J Am Acad Dermatol. 2016;75(4):798–805.e7. https://doi.org/10.1016/j.jaad.2016.06.014.
108. Afifi L, Shankle L, Armstrong AW, Boas M, Bridges A, Chiguil V, et al. National Psoriasis Foundation priorities for patient-centered research: proceedings from the 2016 conference. J Psoriasis Psoriatic Arthritis. 2017;2(3):73–80. https://doi.org/10.1177/247553031700200307.
109. Bell S, Merola JF, Webster DE, Pennington SR, Liao W, Ogdie A, et al. Aiming for cure and preventive initiatives in psoriatic disease: building synergy at NPF, GRAPPA, and PPACMAN. Curr Rheumatol Rep. 2020;22(11):78. https://doi.org/10.1007/s11926-020-00958-9.
110. MINDERA: psoriasis: a chronic disease. https://www.minderadx.com/psoriasis/ (2021). Accessed 11 July 2021.

Psoriasis Biologics and the COVID-19 Pandemic: Lessons Learned

12

Edward Hadeler, Julie Hong, Megan Mosca, Marwa Hakimi, and Tina Bhutani

Introduction

When the World Health Organization declared the coronavirus disease 2019 (COVID-19), caused by the novel severe acute respiratory syndrome coronavirus 2 (SARS-CoV-2), a global pandemic in March 2020, it reported fever, cough, and dyspnea as the most common symptoms of infection [1]. As global understanding of the disease further developed, diarrhea, anosmia, and ageusia were added. In severe cases, it can cause pneumonia, acute respiratory distress syndrome (ARDS), and multiorgan failure. To date, researchers continue to report new manifestations of COVID-19 infection.

The role of biologics being beneficial, neutral, or detrimental in terms of susceptibility to the infection and/or severity of COVID-19 disease is an area of ongoing research [2]. Given their immune-modulating mechanism of action, some concerns have arisen that biologics may increase the risk of COVID-19 infection and potentially cause a more severe course of the disease. Other researchers suggest immune-modulating agents may be beneficial and protective against COVID-19, protecting patients from the severe inflammation [2]. With the implementation of vaccinations for COVID-19, new concerns have arisen over the impact biologics have on vaccination efficacy and safety [3]. Finally, physical distancing requirements early in the pandemic led to the augmentation of new technologies into the dermatology clinic workflow, including teledermatology, which may serve as a desirable option for psoriasis patients on biologic maintenance therapy moving forward.

In this chapter, we discuss data regarding COVID-19 infection risk and outcomes in psoriasis patients on biologics, the role of biologics in treating cytokine storm, data regarding vaccination responses in psoriasis patients on biologics, and the role of teledermatology for psoriasis patients on biologics and its potential use moving forward.

COVID-19 Infection Risk and Outcomes in Psoriasis Patients on Biologics

Because biologics may lead to a slightly increased risk of contracting opportunistic infections, concerns arose over their potential to increase the risk of COVID-19 infection, which became an immediate focal point of research across the world in 2020 [2].

This paper has not been previously published or posted and is not under consideration elsewhere.

E. Hadeler (✉) · J. Hong · M. Mosca · M. Hakimi
University of California, San Francisco, Department of Dermatology, Psoriasis and Skin Treatment Center, San Francisco, CA, USA

T. Bhutani
Department of Dermatology, Psoriasis and Skin Treatment Center, University of California, San Francisco, San Francisco, CA, USA

N. Brownstone et al. (eds.), *Biologic Therapy for Psoriasis*, Updates in Clinical Dermatology,
https://doi.org/10.1007/978-3-030-92938-1_12

To date, large registry studies have reported promising results regarding COVID-19 infection risk of biologic patients. These studies enrolled psoriasis patients who received at least one dose of biologics blocking either tumor necrosis factor (TNF)-alpha, interleukin (IL)-12/23, IL-17, or IL-23 prior to the onset of the pandemic. One of the largest COVID-19 biologic registry studies was conducted by Talamonti et al. They reported data from the PSO-BIO-COVID registry, which included 12,807 psoriasis patients on biologic therapy across 33 Italian dermatology clinics. Of this population, only 26 patients (0.2%) received a confirmed diagnosis of COVID-19 compared to 0.31% of the general Italian population at that time [4]. Overall, the findings of this study suggest that the use of biologics was not associated with a higher risk of COVID-19 infection [5]. Psoriasis patients on biologics were hospitalized at a lower rate and those who were hospitalized had comorbidities and risk factors for severe infection [4, 6, 7], similar to the general population [5].

Other smaller studies from France [6], Turkey [7, 8], and Italy [9–11] presenting real-world [6, 9, 10], retrospective [11], and cross-sectional data [8] also found that biologic use in psoriasis patients did not increase the incidence of infection nor worsen disease course in comparison with the general population [5]. Interestingly, some studies report similar outcomes between psoriasis patients on biologics versus those on other systemic agents, including methotrexate [12]. However, one study reported better outcomes for psoriasis patients on biologics [13]. Specifically, this study compared 374 clinician-reported patients from 25 countries and reported that that patients using nonbiologic systemics had a higher rate of hospitalization due to COVID-19 compared to patients using biologics (OR = 2.84; 95% CI = 1.31–6.18) [13].

One prospective, observational study evaluated COVID-19 infection risk of psoriasis patients on biologics versus those on topicals alone. In this single-center study conducted between January 2020 and May 2020, Brazzelli et al. enrolled 180 patients in Italy (80 patients on topical therapy alone and 100 patients on biologic therapy). The researchers found no statistically significant difference between COVID-19 infection risk and symptom severity between the two groups [14].

The data presented here, including data from observational, retrospective, and cross-sectional studies, show that psoriasis patients treated with biologic agents do not have an increased risk of COVID-19 infection. Despite this, three studies report patients delayed or discontinued treatment during the pandemic, many of whom did so voluntarily without seeking medical advice [7, 15, 16] out of concern for increased fear of infection [7]. Therefore, it is important for providers to educate patients on the causes and risk factors for COVID-19 infection and the importance of seeking medical advice before altering treatment regimens.

Recommendations provided by the American Academy of Dermatology (AAD) and the National Psoriasis Foundation (NPF) COVID-19 Task Force advise that patients not infected with COVID-19 should continue their biologic [17] and should not stop their systemic therapy without consulting physicians [18]. The AAD recommends that physicians discontinue or delay systemic immunosuppressive agents, including biologics, if a patient tests positive for COVID-19 infection or exhibits signs and symptoms of COVID-19 infection [18], though the NPF Task Force states that a final decision should still be determined on a case-by-case basis [17]. Patients who stopped their biologic due to COVID-19 infection are recommended to restart their treatment regimen once they completely recover from COVID-19 based on guidelines provided by the Center for Disease Control and Prevention (CDC) [18]. The CDC recommends persons with COVID-19 who have symptoms isolate at least 10 days after symptom onset and 24 hours since resolution of fever without fever-reducing medications [19]. The use of RT-PCR testing for SARS-CoV-2 RNA to inform discontinuation of isolation should be considered for patients who are severely immunocompromised in consultation with infectious disease experts [19]. For patients considering systemic immunosuppressive agents for the first time, physicians should assess the risks and benefits on a case-by-case basis before initiating any therapy [18].

COVID-19 Vaccination Responses in Patients Receiving Biologics

With the rapid development of vaccines for COVID-19, providers should also be aware of current data discussing the vaccination responses of patients on biologics, to educate and alleviate concerns of patients. Gisondi et al. described the concerns of COVID-19 vaccination in psoriatic patients, highlighting the fact that patients on immunosuppressive therapy were excluded from clinical trials evaluating the efficacy of the COVID-19 vaccination leaving an absence of data on the efficacy of the COVID-19 vaccine for patients treated with biologic agents. Though Gisondi et al. suggest a concern over the reduced effectiveness of the vaccine, they emphasize that having any degree of protection from COVID-19 is better than none [20].

Studies have evaluated factors influencing patients' decision to obtain vaccination [21]. Sotiriou et al. found that psoriasis patients were more likely to obtain vaccination compared to patients without psoriasis. Within psoriasis patients, they identified seven factors associated with an increased likelihood of COVID-19 vaccination: younger age, female sex, higher education, treatment with biologics, history of COPD, diabetes, or malignancy [21]. Among psoriasis patients who were hesitant to obtain COVID-19 vaccination, reasons included the safety and effectiveness of the vaccination (94%), risk of psoriasis flares (21%), and inconvenience of obtaining vaccination (0.8%) [21].

Current data describing the safety regarding the COVID-19 vaccination in psoriasis patients are limited to case series. Damiani et al. reported data on 4 patients with psoriasis who were on biologic therapy who obtained the Pfizer® mRNA vaccination for COVID-19 [3]. Two patients were treated with secukinumab, one patient was treated with ixekizumab and one patient was treated with risankizumab. All four patients experienced no flares after administration of both COVID-19 vaccination doses [3]. Regarding the effectiveness of the vaccination, all patients developed the anti-S1 receptor-binding domain IgG against COVID-19. Ultimately, the cases presented by Damiani et al. suggest the COVID-19 RNA-based vaccine is safe and effective in patients treated with biologic therapies, but larger cohort studies and real-world data are needed to form stronger conclusions.

Reported cutaneous reactions related to the COVID-19 vaccine have included immediate injection site reactions, which were observed in 84.2% of patients after the first dose [22]. Delayed, large, local reactions have also been reported [23–25]. A case series reported this reaction in 12 patients with a median onset of 8 days after the first dose [23]. A subsequent report by Samarakoon et al. reported that 55 of 510 reported delayed, large, local reactions in the COVID-19 vaccine allergy case registry were in patients who were Black, Indigenous, or People of Color [25].

The NPF COVID-19 Task Force recommends the urgent administration of COVID-19 vaccinations to psoriasis patients as soon as it becomes available to them based on federal, state, and local guidelines [17]. They also emphasize that psoriasis patients should continue their biologic and other systemic therapies after receiving the vaccination [17].

In summary, psoriasis patients receiving biologic therapy should receive the COVID-19 vaccination. However, further studies are needed to continue to monitor the safety of the vaccination in this population and the effectiveness of the vaccination doses over time.

Teledermatology for Biologic Monitoring

Though it experienced a resurgence during the COVID-19 pandemic, the use of teledermatology spans decades. Its use showed promise in extending dermatology care to remote populations [26], and some studies even highlighted its effective use in improving clinical outcomes in psoriasis patients [27]. Teledermatology can be implemented primarily through two modalities, live interactive and store and forward [28]. Live interactive involves direct communication between a provider and patient over a live-video interface, like an in-person visit. Store and forward involves the transmission of photographs by a patient, primary care provider, or other healthcare professionals, to a dermatologist for remote evaluation. Physical distancing requirements brought about by the COVID-19 pandemic led to the rapid adoption of teledermatology across dermatology practices in 2020 [29]. To facilitate a smoother transition to the use of teledermatology, many states lifted interstate practice restrictions, allowing physicians to see their patients virtually across state borders if necessary. While physical distancing requirements are expected to be lifted and in-person visits resume, the increased usage of teledermatology was reported to be beneficial for some patients on biologic therapy and may serve as a preferable and convenient option moving forward.

Gisondi et al. evaluated the preference of teledermatology for patients with stable plaque psoriasis on biologic maintenance therapy [30]. Adult patients with chronic plaque psoriasis who were receiving a biologic therapy were surveyed about their preference regarding teledermatology versus in-person visits. A total of 118 (48%) patients stated preference of teledermatology over in-person appointments. Multivariate analysis found that previous experience with digital video-communication tools increased preference for teledermatology, while older age (>60 years) was associated with preference for in-person visits. Reasons for preference of teledermatology were also obtained from patients, and among those interviewed, saving time and safety in relation to COVID-19 risk were some of the most cited. The most common reason for patients to prefer in-person visits was lack of comfort with video-communication tools. Overall, this study demonstrates that for established patients on maintenance therapy, teledermatology may be a convenient and effective option moving forward.

The AAD provides a position statement on the use of teledermatology and states that the consulting dermatologist should (i) have an existing physician–patient relationship, or (ii) establish a physician–patient relationship through live-interactive teledermatology, or (iii) have access to the patient's past and current medical records to enable care coordination [31] prior to initiating follow-up visits through teledermatology.

Lessons Learned and Implications for Future Novel Viral Outbreaks

The COVID-19 pandemic created concerns and fears in the psoriasis patient population, especially in those taking immune-modulating agents, such as biologics. With continuance of the COVID-19 pandemic and the potential onset of future viral outbreaks, many lessons can be learned from the data emerging during this time.

Multiple studies suggest that the use of biologic agents in patients with psoriasis does not increase their risk to COVID-19 infection. Furthermore, psoriasis patients on biologics are not more likely to have severe outcomes of COVID-19 infection and some data suggest patients on biologics may achieve better outcomes compared to patients on nonbiologic systemics. Practitioners should urge patients to seek medical advice before changing or discontinuing therapy during the current pandemic and in the event of future viral outbreaks.

Dermatologists should encourage patients to get vaccinated as soon as possible. Provision of evidence-based information regarding COVID-19 and the safety of vaccines to patients is essential.

The COVID-19 pandemic led to emergence of technologies to facilitate remote care. Psoriasis patients managed with biologics who have stable disease should be presented with the option to receive follow-up care through teledermatology.

References

1. Huang C, Wang Y, Li X, Ren L, Zhao J, Hu Y, et al. Clinical features of patients infected with 2019 novel coronavirus in Wuhan, China. Lancet. 2020;395(10223):497–506.

2. Amerio P, Prignano F, Giuliani F, Gualdi G. COVID-19 and psoriasis: should we fear for patients treated with biologics? Dermatol Ther. 2020;33(4):e13434.
3. Damiani G, Allocco F, Young Dermatologists Italian Network, Malagoli P. COVID-19 vaccination and patients with psoriasis under biologics: real-life evidence on safety and effectiveness from Italian vaccinated healthcare workers. Clin Exp Dermatol. 2021;46(6):1106–8.
4. Talamonti M, Galluzzo M, Chiricozzi A, Quaglino P, Fabbrocini G, Gisondi P, et al. Characteristic of chronic plaque psoriasis patients treated with biologics in Italy during the COVID-19 pandemic: risk analysis from the PSO-BIO-COVID observational study. Expert Opin Biol Ther. 2021;21(2):271–7.
5. Italian Institute of Health Report [Internet]. Available from: https://www.epicentro.iss.it/en/coronavirus/bollettino/Report-COVID-2019_23_april_2020.pdf
6. Fougerousse A-C, Perrussel M, Bécherel P-A, Begon E, Pallure V, Zaraa I, et al. Systemic or biologic treatment in psoriasis patients does not increase the risk of a severe form of COVID-19. J Eur Acad Dermatol Venereol. 2020;34(11):e676–9.
7. Polat Ekinci A, Pehlivan G, Gökalp MO. Surveillance of psoriatic patients on biologic treatment during the COVID-19 pandemic: a single-center experience. Dermatol Ther. 2021;34(1):e14700.
8. Kartal SP, Çelik G, Yılmaz O, Öksüm Solak E, Demirbağ Gül B, Üstünbaş TK, et al. The impact of COVID-19 pandemic on psoriasis patients, and their immunosuppressive treatment: a cross-sectional multicenter study from Turkey. J Dermatol Treat. 2021;1–8
9. Vispi M, Corradin T, Peccianti C, Feci L, Casini L, Pisani C, et al. Psoriasis, biological drugs and coronavirus disease 2019: real life experience of two Italian provinces. Dermatol Rep. 2020;12(1):8642.
10. Piaserico S, Gisondi P, Cazzaniga S, Naldi L. Lack of Evidence for an Increased Risk of Severe COVID-19 in Psoriasis Patients on Biologics: A Cohort Study from Northeast Italy. Am J Clin Dermatol [Internet]. 2020 [cited 22 July 2021]; Available from: http://link.springer.com/10.1007/s40257-020-00552-w.
11. Gisondi P, Piaserico S, Naldi L, Dapavo P, Conti A, Malagoli P, et al. Incidence rates of hospitalization and death from COVID-19 in patients with psoriasis receiving biological treatment: a Northern Italy experience. J Allergy Clin Immunol. 2021;147(2):558–560.e1.
12. Kridin K, Schonmann Y, Solomon A, Damiani G, Tzur Bitan D, Onn E, et al. Risk of COVID-19 infection, hospitalization, and mortality in patients with psoriasis treated by interleukin-17 inhibitors. J Dermatolog Treat. 2021;1–28
13. Mahil SK, Dand N, Mason KJ, Yiu ZZN, Tsakok T, Meynell F, et al. Factors associated with adverse COVID-19 outcomes in patients with psoriasis-insights from a global registry-based study. J Allergy Clin Immunol. 2021;147(1):60–71.
14. Brazzelli V, Isoletta E, Barak O, Barruscotti S, Vassallo C, Giorgini C, et al. Does therapy with biological drugs influence COVID-19 infection? Observational monocentric prevalence study on the clinical and epidemiological data of psoriatic patients treated with biological drugs or with topical drugs alone. Dermatol Ther. 2020;33(6):e14516.
15. Camela E, Fabbrocini G, Cinelli E, Lauro W, Megna M. Biologic therapies, psoriasis, and COVID-19: our experience at the psoriasis unit of the University of Naples Federico II. Dermatology. 2021;237(1):13–4.
16. Bragazzi NL, Riccò M, Pacifico A, Malagoli P, Kridin K, Pigatto P, et al. COVID-19 knowledge prevents biologics discontinuation: data from an Italian multicenter survey during RED-ZONE declaration. Dermatol Ther. 2020;33(4):e13508.
17. Gelfand JM, Armstrong AW, Bell S, Anesi GL, Blauvelt A, Calabrese C, et al. National Psoriasis Foundation COVID-19 Task Force guidance for management of psoriatic disease during the pandemic: Version 2—advances in psoriatic disease management, COVID-19 vaccines, and COVID-19 treatments. J Am Acad Dermatol. 2021;84(5):1254–68.
18. American Academy of Dermatology Work Group. Guidance on the use of immunosuppressive agents [Internet]. Available from: https://www.aad.org/member/practice/coronavirus/clinical-guidance/biologics.
19. Ending home isolation for persons with COVID-19 not in healthcare settings [Internet]. Available from: https://www.cdc.gov/coronavirus/2019-ncov/hcp/disposition-in-home-patients.html.
20. Gisondi P, Geat D, Naldi L, Piaserico S. Insights into Sars-CoV-2 vaccination in patients with chronic plaque psoriasis on systemic treatments. J Eur Acad Dermatol Venereol. 2021;35(6):e361–2.
21. Sotiriou E, Bakirtzi K, Papadimitriou I, Paschou E, Vakirlis E, Lallas A, et al. COVID-19 vaccination intention among patients with psoriasis compared with immunosuppressed patients with other skin diseases and factors influencing their decision. Br J Dermatol. 2021;185(1):209–10.
22. Baden LR, El Sahly HM, Essink B, Kotloff K, Frey S, Novak R, et al. Efficacy and safety of the mRNA-1273 SARS-CoV-2 vaccine. N Engl J Med. 2021;384(5):403–16.
23. Blumenthal KG, Freeman EE, Saff RR, Robinson LB, Wolfson AR, Foreman RK, et al. Delayed large local reactions to mRNA-1273 vaccine against SARS-CoV-2. N Engl J Med. 2021;384(13):1273–7.
24. Baeck M, Marot L, Belkhir L. Delayed large local reactions to mRNA vaccines. N Engl J Med. 2021;384(24):e98.
25. Samarakoon U, Alvarez-Arango S, Blumenthal KG. Delayed large local reactions to mRNA Covid-19 vaccines in blacks, indigenous persons, and people of color. N Engl J Med. 2021;385(7):662–4.
26. Norton SA, Burdick AE, Phillips CM, Berman B. Teledermatology and underserved populations. Arch Dermatol. 1997;133(2):197–200.

27. Armstrong AW, Chambers CJ, Maverakis E, Cheng MY, Dunnick CA, Chren M-M, et al. Effectiveness of online vs in-person care for adults with Psoriasis: a randomized clinical trial. JAMA Netw Open. 2018;1(6):e183062.
28. Pasquali P, Sonthalia S, Moreno-Ramirez D, Sharma P, Agrawal M, Gupta S, et al. Teledermatology and its current perspective. Indian Dermatol Online J. 2020;11(1):12–20.
29. The Dermatologist. COVID-19 and teledermatology: the past, present, and future [Internet]. Available from: https://www.the-dermatologist.com/article/covid-19-and-teledermatology-past-present-future.
30. Gisondi P, Bellinato F, Piaserico S, Di Leo S, Cazzaniga S, Naldi L. Preference for telemedicine versus in-person visit among patients with psoriasis receiving biological drugs. Dermatol Ther (Heidelb) [Internet]. 2021 [cited 22 July 2021]; Available from: https://link.springer.com/10.1007/s13555-021-00555-3
31. American Academy of Dermatology Work Group. Position statement on teledermatology [Internet]. Available from: https://server.aad.org/Forms/Policies/Uploads/PS/PS-Teledermatology.pdf?

Adherence to Biologic Therapy for Psoriasis

13

Qisi Sun, Patrick O. Perche, Varun K. Ranpariya, and Steven R. Feldman

Introduction

Approximately 125 million individuals, comprising 2–3% of the world's population, are affected by psoriasis [1]. Although initially thought to be a disorder of epidermal hyperproliferation, psoriasis is now understood to involve the immune system as well, with substantial evidence over the past few decades implicating various immunological pathways and molecules in its pathogenesis. This has led to more specific, targeted therapies such as biologics, adding to the arsenal of standard treatment options such as phototherapy, topical therapeutics, and oral systemic agents.

Biologics are large molecular weight proteins that target immune or genetic mediators involved in psoriasis pathophysiology. Currently, there are 11 Food and Drug Administration (FDA)-approved biologics with many more in the pipeline. These drugs target IL-12/23, IL-23, IL-17, and TNF-α, must be injected and are more suitable for long-term use given their better safety profiles compared to other psoriasis medications [2–4].

While these agents have revolutionized psoriasis treatment and prognosis, they are only as effective as patients' willingness to adhere to their treatment regimen and therapeutic goals. In fact, the World Health Organization (WHO) recognized adherence as one of the key factors influencing psoriasis treatment efficacy [5]. Sometimes used interchangeably with compliance, adherence is defined as the extent to which an individual's behavior corresponds with the therapeutic plan mutually agreed upon by the patient and healthcare provider [5, 6].

Despite experiencing significant comorbidities and burden on quality of life, psoriasis patients have low rates of medication adherence [7]. A 10% decrease in adherence rate is associated with a one-point increase in disease severity on a nine-point scale [8]. In this chapter, we will first discuss objective measures and determinants of adherence, followed by a summary of the current data on adherence to biologics before concluding with a discussion of strategies to improve adherence.

Measures of Adherence

There is no standardized measurement of adherence in real-world settings, and studies to date have utilized a variety of methods (Table 13.1). The most common measure is drug survival, which is the length of time from drug initiation to

Q. Sun (✉)
Department of Dermatology, Yale University School of Medicine, New Haven, CT, USA
e-mail: sfeldman@wakehealth.edu

P. O. Perche · V. K. Ranpariya · S. R. Feldman
Center for Dermatology Research, Wake Forest School of Medicine, Winston-Salem, NC, USA

N. Brownstone et al. (eds.), *Biologic Therapy for Psoriasis*, Updates in Clinical Dermatology,
https://doi.org/10.1007/978-3-030-92938-1_13

Table 13.1 Methods to measure adherence [63]

Type	Definition	Advantages	Disadvantages
Drug survival	Length of time from initiation to drug discontinuation	Simple calculation method	Lack of standardized or uniform definition
Medication possession ratio (MPR)	Number of days a patient has the medication divided by the number of days a patient is eligible to have the medication	Simple calculation method	Difficult to use for large population analysis; does not consider gaps in refills
Proportion of days covered (PDC)	Number of days a patient is covered by the medication divided by the number of days the patient is eligible to have a medication	More specific than MPR	Better quantifies persistence than adherence
Persistence	The absence of prescription refill gaps during usage of a medication		
Group-based trajectory modeling	The utilization of pharmacy dispensing data to measure adherence	Analysis of large population; can identify multidrug adherence; help identify patients at risk of treatment failure	Prescriptions may be missed if obtained outside of insurance plan
Medication event monitoring system (MEMS)	Electronic monitoring system that utilizes a computer chip inserted into a prescription pill bottle cap to recording opening of medication	Reference standard for adherence measurement, highly accurate in several studies; can help identify whether nonadherence is sporadic or consistent; quantifies daily doses	Expensive; bulky container; some patients report anxiety over "constant" surveillance

drug discontinuation [9]. Other methods include self-reports and medication possession ratio (MPR), which evaluates drug access by dividing the number of days a patient has their medicine by the number of days a patient is eligible to have that medicine. While this may not take into account whether the patient is taking the medication as directed, drug access is still an important component of adherence. Some studies utilized proportion of days covered (PDC), defined as the number of days a patient is covered by the medication divided by the number of days the patient is eligible to have the medication. PDC is more specific than MPR, which can sometimes be elevated if the patient picks up his or her medication days in advance. Persistence, defined as the absence of prescription refill gaps during usage of a biologic and group-based trajectory modeling (GBTM), which utilizes pharmacy dispensing data to measure adherence, is additional method [10, 11]. However, defining persistence consistently is challenging given the heterogeneity of dosing regimens across different medications. The Morisky Medication Adherence Scale (MMAS-8) is a self-report measure of medication-taking behavior with a version modified for psoriasis [12]. Electronic monitoring systems such as the Medication Event Monitoring System (MEMS), which involves a computer chip inserted into the prescription pill bottle cap to monitor opening, are also a popular method of adherence evaluation.

Determinants of Adherence to Biologics in Psoriasis Treatment

Factors impacting adherence to biologics among patients with psoriasis can be divided into three main categories: patient-centered, medication-related, and provider-centered.

Patient-Centered Factors

Patients with psoriasis frequently have comorbidities such as psoriatic arthritis (PsA), Crohn's disease (CD), and metabolic syndrome [13]. Some of these concomitant disorders influence adherence to biologics. Individuals with PsA, for instance, tend to have greater rates of drug survival compared to those with only psoriasis [4, 14]. In addition, grasping the consequences associated with severe psoriasis, such as cardiovascular disease, also drives adherence [15]. An absence of comorbidities in general is independently associated with longer drug survival (Table 13.2) [16].

Negative predictors of adherence include concomitant anxiety and obesity [4, 14, 17–22]. A high body mass index (BMI) leads to poor adherence likely because biologics tend to exhibit compromised efficacy among heavier individuals [14, 18, 19, 23–25]. Comorbid metabolic syndrome, on the other hand, has both positive and negative influences on adherence and drug survival [4, 21]. Other negative predictors of adherence include current smoking status and better quality of life as assessed by the Dermatology Life Quality Index (DLQI) (Table 13.2) [26].

Table 13.2 Determinants of biologic adherence

Positive determinants	Reference(s)
PsA	[4, 14]
Knowledge of comorbidities associated with severe psoriasis	[15]
Absence of comorbidities	[16]
Comorbid metabolic syndrome	[21]
PASI-75 score	[34–36]
Failure of previous biologic therapy if the current biologic is sufficiently effective	[4, 15, 26, 64]
Combination treatment	[30, 38]
Ustekinumab	[14, 16, 20, 27, 36, 37, 43, 44, 48, 53, 65]
Negative determinants	
Concomitant anxiety	[10, 12, 17]
Elevated BMI/obesity	[14, 17–22, 38]
Comorbid metabolic syndrome	[4]
Current smoking status	[26]
High DLQI	[26]
Age (<65, >75 years)	[27]
Low socioeconomic status and medication costs	[21, 27, 37]
Female sex	[14, 16, 21, 22, 27, 29, 30]
AEs	[14, 16, 31–33]
Therapeutic inefficacy	[14, 16, 31, 33]
Prior biologic therapy	[9, 34]

Patient demographics and characteristics also influence adherence. In a study of US Medicare psoriasis patients receiving biologics, individuals younger than 65 years or older than 75 years tended to be less adherent [27]. Age was only moderately correlated with adherence in another study, which utilized the MMAS-8; older patients were more adherent than younger patients. A high socioeconomic status is also associated with increased biologic drug survival [21]. However, when comparing medication adherence of white versus non-white patients, race did not have a large effect on MPR or PDC [27, 28]. The female sex tends to be a predictor of decreased adherence or early discontinuation of biologics, and this pattern is also seen in the treatment of hypertension and post-myocardial infarction (Table 13.2) [14, 16, 27, 29, 30]. It is unclear whether this is due to healthcare delivery inequities or differences in biology, but one possible explanation for this observation is that women tend to have a higher rate of severe adverse events (AEs), which may encourage drug discontinuation [14].

Medication-Related Factors

Side effects and therapeutic ineffectiveness are the most common medication-related factors contributing to nonadherence (Table 13.2) [14, 16, 31–33]. Biologics are associated with a variety of AEs such as injection site reactions, infections, infusion reactions, lupus-like symptoms, tuberculosis (TB) reactivation, and malignancy [32]. Although these side effects are uncommon, they can still promote patient reluctance to use these agents. Furthermore, the risk of these AEs is higher among patients treated intermittently rather than continuously with biologics. Treatment inefficacy and loss of response over time also engender patient frustration and promote nonadherence. In contrast, treatment-related disease improvement as measured by a 75% reduction in Psoriasis Area and Severity Index (PASI-75) was associated with increased adherence to certain biologics [34–36]. Failure of preceding biologic therapy can also promote adherence to the current biologic medication if the latter is sufficiently effective [4, 15, 26]. However, prior exposure to biologics may compromise the efficacy of subsequent biologic medications, and a biologic-naive status is associated with prolonged biologic drug survival [9, 11, 34].

Other medication-related factors impacting adherence include drug affordability, insurance coverage issues, and combination treatment [37, 38]. High costs and problems with coverage have been cited as one of the major reasons for missed doses of ustekinumab [37]. Similarly, patients receiving biologics who faced significant cost sharing under Medicare Part D were also more likely to be treatment nonadherent [27]. Individuals treated with a combination of medications, such as methotrexate with infliximab, had longer drug survival rates compared to those treated solely with infliximab (Table 13.2) [38]. This is likely because combination treatment inhibits the formation of anti-drug antibodies, thus leading to better efficacy and drug survival [38].

Provider-Centered Factors

The very definition of adherence extends beyond merely following physician orders. According to one study, most psoriasis patients attributed their reasons for biologic discontinuation to their dermatologist rather than a joint decision [15]. Although the sample size in that study was small, the finding suggests that more physician–patient communication is needed and can improve patient adherence. Physicians may also prescribe expensive medications that patients cannot afford or fail to set expectations, adequately explain possible side effects, or provide an efficient means for which patients can communicate with their doctors in case of unforeseen challenges. To promote adherence, a positive patient–physician relationship and a frank discussion of the patient's goals and lifestyle are warranted. This will enable the creation of a treatment plan that allows for optimal convenience for the patient [15, 39].

Adherence Associated with Biologic Treatments

Not all biologics are created equal with regard to associated adherence and drug survival, which decreases over time (Table 13.3) [40, 41]. Awareness of these differences can help providers determine the most appropriate biologic for each patient to optimize adherence.

Table 13.3 Adherence and dosing of biologics

Biologic	Adherence	Dosing
Ustekinumab	90% adherence at 3 years measured by drug survival [44] 83.7% adherence [45] 83% adherence at 3 years measured by drug survival [49] 79.4% adherence measured by drug survival at 1 year [48] 22% adherence at 2 years measured by PDC [41] 81.8% adherence at 1 year measured by MPR (MPR > 0.80%) [42] 50.6% adherence at 1 year measured by PDC (PDC > 0.80%) [42] 56% adherence at 4 years measured by drug survival [40] 96.7% adherence at 1 year measured by drug survival [53] 89% adherence at 1 year measured by drug survival [14]	Two initial 45 mg loading doses with 45 mg maintenance doses every 12 weeks thereafter

Table 13.3 (continued)

Biologic	Adherence	Dosing
Etanercept	80.7% adherence over average observation period of 28.9 ± 15.4 months measured by drug survival [30] 38% adherence at 3 years measured by drug survival [49] MPR adherence score of 0.94 (>0.8 considered "very good") but lower than adalimumab and ustekinumab (1.0 & 1.0 respectively) [47] 55.5% adherence at 1 year measured by drug survival [48] 40% adherence at 4 years measured by drug survival [29] 50% adherence at 4 years measured by drug survival [44] 19.6% adherence at 2 years measured by PDC [41] 56.4% adherence at 1 year measured by MPR (MPR > 0.80%) [42] 19.5% adherence at 1 year measured by PDC (PDC > 0.80%) [42] 41% adherence at 4 years measured by drug survival [40] 70% adherence at 1 year measured by drug survival [14]	50 mg doses twice weekly for the first 12 weeks and 50 mg once weekly thereafter
Adalimumab	49% adherence at 3 years measured by drug survival [49] 64.6% adherence at 1 year measured by drug survival [48] 40% adherence measured at 4 years measured by drug survival [29] 40% adherence at 4 years measured by drug survival [44] 26.5% adherence at 2 years measured by PDC [41] 67.9% adherence at 1 year measured by MPR (MPR > 0.80%) [42] 35.6% adherence at 1 year measured by PDC (PDC > 0.80%) [42] 47% adherence at 4 years measured by drug survival [40] 79.7% adherence at 1 year measured by drug survival [53] 59% adherence at 5 years measured by drug survival [34] 79% adherence at 1 year measured by drug survival [14]	Two initial 40 mg loading doses at weeks 0 and 1 with 40 mg maintenance doses every 2 weeks thereafter

(continued)

Table 13.3 (continued)

Biologic	Adherence	Dosing
Infliximab	37% adherence at 3 years measured by drug survival [49] 63.6% adherence at 1 year measured by drug survival [48] 70% adherence at 4 years measured by drug survival [29] 50% adherence at 4 years measured by drug survival [44] 42% adherence at 4 years measured by drug survival [40] 73.3% adherence at 1 year measured by drug survival [53] 61.9% adherence over average observation period of 28.9 ± 15.4 months measured by drug survival [30] 65% adherence at 1 year measured by drug survival [14]	5 mg/kg/dose at 0, 2, and 6 weeks, and then at 8–12 week intervals thereafter
Secukinumab	36.1% adherence at 2 years measured by PDC [41] 68% adherence at 1 year measured by MPR (MPR > 0.80%) [42] 41.7% adherence at 1 year measured by PDC (PDC > 0.80%) [42] 45% adherence at 2 years measured by drug survival [54]	Initial 300 mg dose at weeks 0, 1, 2, 3, and 4 followed by maintenance dose every 4 weeks thereafter

Ustekinumab

Although ustekinumab is less efficacious compared to newer agents, it has higher rates of adherence and drug survival and lower rates of discontinuation compared to other biologics [11, 41, 42]. For instance, during an observation period of 1 year, patients treated with ustekinumab had excellent adherence compared to those treated with adalimumab or etanercept, despite similar baseline characteristics [43]. Ustekinumab emerged again as the biologic with the greatest adherence in a prospective case review of patients receiving etanercept, adalimumab, infliximab, and ustekinumab [44]. After 3 years, 90% of these patients on ustekinumab were still adherent and were 6.7-fold less likely to discontinue treatment compared to those on etanercept [44]. In a single-center study, ustekinumab had an average adherence rate of 83.7% [45]. These findings may be attributable to ustekinumab's superior efficacy, low immunogenicity, tolerable side effect profile, and convenient administration schedule, as only four maintenance injections are required each year. In addition, previous failure to biologics, particularly TNF-α inhibitors, did not compromise response to subsequent ustekinumab treatment, suggesting that ustekinumab may be an ideal choice for patients who experienced little to no disease improvement with anti-TNF-α medications [43].

The TNF-α Inhibitors

Etanercept

Etanercept not only has one of the best FDA "geriatric statements" testifying to its safety in elderly patients, but it is also approved for use in children age 4 years and older [46]. In addition, it has the lowest risk of TB reactivation compared to the other two TNF-α inhibitors, adalimumab and infliximab [46].

Etanercept tended to have lower rates of drug survival and adherence compared to other drugs such as adalimumab, infliximab, methotrexate, and ustekinumab [29, 47, 48]. However, in one study, etanercept had a higher drug survival than infliximab and methotrexate, and in two other investigations, etanercept was observed to have a higher drug survival rate than infliximab and adalimumab [30, 49, 50]. These contradictory findings may be due to differences in study design, as some did not mention whether etanercept was used intermittently or whether the analysis was limited to biologic-naive patients [30].

Unlike ustekinumab, etanercept's drug survival rate was lower in those who had previously been treated with biologics [49]. Providers should balance these considerations with etanercept's excellent safety profile in the pediatric and elderly populations in order to optimize treatment efficacy and adherence.

Adalimumab

In general, adherence to adalimumab is very variable and can be poor [51]. In some studies, adalimumab survival rates were greater than that of etanercept and infliximab [29, 40]. In another study, adalimumab survival rates were lower than etanercept but higher than that of infliximab, although the differences were insignificant [52]. In other investigations, only 50.8% of 59 patients treated with adalimumab achieved PASI-75, an efficacy rate lower that of ustekinumab and infliximab [53]. Furthermore, in a different study with a cohort of 119 psoriasis patients treated with adalimumab, 49 individuals (41%) discontinued the medication mainly due to drug inefficacy and AEs [34]. Given the advantages of combination therapy, the addition of other treatments to adalimumab may increase adherence and efficacy.

Infliximab

Infliximab is associated with infusion reactions, cancer, and infections—AEs that predicted decreased drug survival [38]. In general, infliximab drug survival rates were comparable to that of adalimumab and similarly variable from study to study [11, 14, 29, 30]. Although AEs are generally uncommon among biologics, infliximab was associated with greater side effects and higher rates of discontinuation [32]. US dermatologists in general rarely use infliximab, especially with newer and more efficacious biologics available in the arsenal.

Secukinumab

Although secukinumab has superior efficacy compared to other biologics such as etanercept and ustekinumab, its adherence rate is variable and suboptimal. One study revealed that 68% of patients receiving secukinumab had an MPR greater than or equal to 80%, and 41.7% had a PDC greater than or equal to 80% [42]. In two recent studies, secukinumab had the lowest drug survival and highest discontinuation rates compared to etanercept, infliximab, adalimumab, and ustekinumab [41, 46, 54].

Current literature investigating adherence to other biologics such as risankizumab, guselkumab, brodalumab, tildrakizumab, ixekizumab, apremilast, and certolizumab is limited.

Strategies to Enhance Adherence to Biologic Treatments in Psoriasis

A tailored, patient-centered approach is critical to enhancing adherence to biologics. Overall, patients noted that treatment efficacy and AEs were the two most important factors influencing their decision to adhere to a medication [55]. However, patient preferences varied. For instance, men were more concerned than women about treatment efficacy, while women were more concerned about the convenience of the dosing schedule [55]. Similarly, older individuals attached more value to treatment efficacy and side effect tolerability than younger individuals [55]. In addition, those who worked full time were more concerned about treatment efficacy, time to response, and dosing schedule than those who worked part time [55]. Therefore, an effective patient–provider relationship and a thorough discussion of treatment goals, expectations, and concerns are necessary to promote optimal adherence.

Accountability is another powerful tool that should be leveraged to improve treatment adherence. Defined as the "expectation of account-giving" involving an expected social interaction, accountability is rarely used in real-world clinical practice [56]. For instance, many patients are initiated on a new medication with no follow-up until months later. The lack of anticipation of frequent social interactions between patient and provider during this time may discourage adherence. In fact, patient adherence increases before consultations and decreases between visits, a phenomenon called "white coat compliance" and similar to the Hawthorne effect, in which individuals modify their behavior because they know they are being observed [57–59]. Therefore, early follow-up visits after initiation of a new biologic are important. Direct human contact is not always necessary, however. According to one study, patients who received daily electronic reminders experienced an increase in adherence and quality of life compared to those who did not (Table 13.4) [60]. Therefore, text reminders, accountability partners, and weekly online reporting are ways to implement accountability in real-world settings at a low cost [56].

Other techniques include anchoring, patient education, and history evaluation. Anchoring is defined as the tendency for humans to make decisions relative to the initial piece of information presented [61]. For instance, providers can first assess a patient's willingness to start a once-daily injectable biologic and then follow-up by asking about their willingness to take the medication if it only requires a once-monthly injection [61]. Anchoring increases a patient's willingness to take an injectable biologic [61]. Reframing of the risk of adverse events may also allay lingering fears. For instance, a 1% chance of an AE can be explained as a 99% chance of no AE occurrence [62]. Also essential to adherence are patient education on injection technique and a discussion of the consequences of severe, untreated psoriasis. Lastly, since the choice of biologic impacts adherence, an evaluation of the patient's past medical history, such as their satisfaction with previous treatments, if any, is warranted to allow appropriate biologic selection (Table 13.4).

Table 13.4 Adherence interventions

Strategies to augment adherence	References
Treatment regimen tailored to patient preference	[55, 66]
Early follow-up visits	[57–59, 67]
Electronic/phone reminders	[60, 68]
Anchoring	[61, 67]
Reframing risks	[62, 67]
Patient education and medical history evaluation	[11, 15]

Conclusion

The advent of biologics has heralded a new chapter in psoriasis treatment. Despite their effectiveness, adherence to these medications remains suboptimal and discontinuation is common [41]. Poor medication adherence not only leads to adverse health outcomes but also increased financial expenditure since the cost of induction for biologics is higher than that of maintenance [38].

Ustekinumab consistently emerged as the biologic with the highest adherence and lowest drug discontinuation rate. The data for other biologics varied across studies, likely due to differences in study design, thus attesting to a need for standardization of adherence measures. Furthermore, limitations exist when comparing the adherence of multiple biologics due to variations in dosing schedules. Many factors influence a patient's decision to not adhere to the treatment plan or discontinue a drug, some of which include therapeutic inefficacy, loss of response over time, AEs, poor socioeconomic status, and costs. An individualized plan shaped to the patient's goals, preferences, and disease condition can augment adherence and improve clinical outcomes. This ideal, in turn, can only be achieved through a strong patient–physician relationship, with both parties committed to establishing trust, gaining a mutual understanding of beliefs and expectations, and addressing challenges early.

References

1. Foundation NP. Psoriasis statistics. https://www.psoriasis.org/psoriasis-statistics/#:~:text=Prevalence&text=1%5D-,125%20million%20people%20worldwide%E2%80%942%20to%203%20percent%20of%20the,the%20World%20Psoriasis%20Day%20consortium. (2020). Accessed 1 Apr 2021.
2. Bakshi H, Nagpal M, Singh M, Dhingra GA, Aggarwal G. Treatment of psoriasis: a comprehensive review of entire therapies. Curr Drug Saf. 2020;15(2):82–104. https://doi.org/10.2174/157488631566620012809595 8.
3. Rendon A, Schäkel K. Psoriasis pathogenesis and treatment. Int J Mol Sci. 2019;20(6):1475. https://doi.org/10.3390/ijms20061475.
4. Jacobi A, Rustenbach SJ, Augustin M. Comorbidity as a predictor for drug survival of biologic therapy in patients with psoriasis. Int J Dermatol. 2016;55(3):296–302. https://doi.org/10.1111/ijd.12879.
5. World Health Organization. Adherence to long term therapy: evidence for action. 2003. https://www.who.int/chp/knowledge/publications/adherence_full_report.pdf. Accessed 30 Mar 2021.
6. Augustin M, Holland B, Dartsch D, Langenbruch A, Radtke MA. Adherence in the treatment of psoriasis: a systematic review. Dermatology. 2011;222(4):363–74. https://doi.org/10.1159/000329026.
7. Storm A, Andersen SE, Benfeldt E, Serup J. One in 3 prescriptions are never redeemed: primary nonadherence in an outpatient clinic. J Am Acad Dermatol. 2008;59(1):27–33. https://doi.org/10.1016/j.jaad.2008.03.045.
8. Carroll CL, Feldman SR, Camacho FT, Balkrishnan R. Better medication adherence results in greater improvement in severity of psoriasis. Br J Dermatol. 2004;151(4):895–7. https://doi.org/10.1111/j.1365-2133.2004.06174.x.
9. No DJ, Inkeles MS, Amin M, Wu JJ. Drug survival of biologic treatments in psoriasis: a systematic review. J Dermatolog Treat. 2018;29(5):460–6. https://doi.org/10.1080/09546634.2017.1398393.
10. Dillon P, Stewart D, Smith SM, Gallagher P, Cousins G. Group-based trajectory models: assessing adherence to antihypertensive medication in older adults in a community pharmacy setting. Clin Pharmacol Ther. 2018;103(6):1052–60. https://doi.org/10.1002/cpt.865.
11. Seale L, Cardwell LA, Feldman SR. Adherence to biologics in patients with psoriasis. Expert Rev Clin Immunol. 2018;14(2):155–61. https://doi.org/10.1080/1744666x.2018.1427065.
12. Hambly R, Kelly A, Gilhooley E, Nic Dhonncha E, Murad A, Hughes R, et al. Medication adherence among patients with psoriasis on traditional systemic and biologics treatment. Br J Dermatol. 2018;178(1):e46–e8. https://doi.org/10.1111/bjd.15856.
13. Oliveira MFSP, Rocha BO, Duarte GV. Psoriasis: classical and emerging comorbidities. An Bras Dermatol. 2015;90(1):9–20. https://doi.org/10.1590/abd1806-4841.20153038.
14. Warren RB, Smith CH, Yiu ZZN, Ashcroft DM, Barker JNWN, Burden AD, et al. Differential drug survival of biologic therapies for the treatment of psoriasis: a prospective observational cohort study from the British Association of Dermatologists Biologic Interventions Register (BADBIR). J Investig Dermatol. 2015;135(11):2632–40. https://doi.org/10.1038/jid.2015.208.
15. Zschocke I, Ortland C, Reich K. Evaluation of adherence predictors for the treatment of moderate to severe psoriasis with biologics: the importance of physician–patient interaction and communication. J Eur Acad Dermatol Venereol. 2017;31(6):1014–20. https://doi.org/10.1111/jdv.14178.
16. van den Reek JMPA, Tummers M, Zweegers J, Seyger MMB, van Lümig PPM, Driessen RJB, et al. Predictors of adalimumab drug survival in psoriasis differ by reason for discontinuation: long-term results from the Bio-CAPTURE registry. J Eur Acad Dermatol Venereol. 2015;29(3):560–5. https://doi.org/10.1111/jdv.12636.
17. Murage MJ, Tongbram V, Feldman SR, Malatestinic WN, Larmore CJ, Muram TM, et al. Medication adherence and persistence in patients with rheumatoid arthritis, psoriasis, and psoriatic arthritis: a systematic literature review. Patient Prefer Adherence. 2018;12:1483–503. https://doi.org/10.2147/PPA.S167508.
18. Carrascosa JM, Vilavella M, Garcia-Doval I, Carretero G, Vanaclocha F, Daudén E, et al. Body mass index in patients with moderate-to-severe psoriasis in Spain and its impact as an independent risk factor for therapy withdrawal: results of the Biobadaderm Registry. J Eur Acad Dermatol Venereol. 2014;28(7):907–14. https://doi.org/10.1111/jdv.12208.
19. Di Lernia V, Tasin L, Pellicano R, Zumiani G, Albertini G. Impact of body mass index on retention rates of anti-TNF-alfa drugs in daily practice for psoriasis. J Dermatol Treat. 2012;23(6):404–9. https://doi.org/10.3109/09546634.2011.593489.
20. Vilarrasa E, Notario J, Bordas X, López-Ferrer A, Gich IJ, Puig L. ORBIT (outcome and retention rate of biologic treatments for psoriasis): a retrospective observational study on biologic drug survival in daily practice. J Am Acad Dermatol. 2016;74(6):1066–72. https://doi.org/10.1016/j.jaad.2016.01.037.
21. Shalom G, Cohen AD, Ziv M, Eran CB, Feldhamer I, Freud T, et al. Biologic drug survival in Israeli psoriasis patients. J Am Acad Dermatol. 2017;76(4):662–9.e1. https://doi.org/10.1016/j.jaad.2016.10.033.
22. Zweegers J, van den Reek JM, van de Kerkhof PC, Otero ME, Kuijpers AL, Koetsier MI, et al. Body

mass index predicts discontinuation due to ineffectiveness and female sex predicts discontinuation due to side-effects in patients with psoriasis treated with adalimumab, etanercept or ustekinumab in daily practice: a prospective, comparative, long-term drug-survival study from the BioCAPTURE registry. Br J Dermatol. 2016;175(2):340–7. https://doi.org/10.1111/bjd.14552.
23. Kisielnicka A, Szczerkowska-Dobosz A, Nowicki RJ. The influence of body weight of patients with chronic plaque psoriasis on biological treatment response. Postepy Dermatol Alergol. 2020;37(2):168–73. https://doi.org/10.5114/ada.2020.94835.
24. Naldi L, Addis A, Chimenti S, Giannetti A, Picardo M, Tomino C, et al. Impact of body mass index and obesity on clinical response to systemic treatment for psoriasis. Dermatology. 2008;217(4):365–73. https://doi.org/10.1159/000156599.
25. Edson-Heredia E, Sterling KL, Alatorre CI, Cuyun Carter G, Paczkowski R, Zarotsky V, et al. Heterogeneity of response to biologic treatment: perspective for psoriasis. J Investig Dermatol. 2014;134(1):18–23. https://doi.org/10.1038/jid.2013.326.
26. Chan SA, Hussain F, Lawson LG, Ormerod AD. Factors affecting adherence to treatment of psoriasis: comparing biologic therapy to other modalities. J Dermatolog Treat. 2013;24(1):64–9. https://doi.org/10.3109/09546634.2011.607425.
27. Doshi JA, Takeshita J, Pinto L, Li P, Yu X, Rao P, et al. Biologic therapy adherence, discontinuation, switching, and restarting among patients with psoriasis in the US Medicare population. J Am Acad Dermatol. 2016;74(6):1057–65.e4. https://doi.org/10.1016/j.jaad.2016.01.048.
28. Bhosle MJ, Feldman SR, Camacho FT, Timothy Whitmire J, Nahata MC, Balkrishnan R. Medication adherence and health care costs associated with biologics in Medicaid-enrolled patients with psoriasis. J Dermatolog Treat. 2006;17(5):294–301. https://doi.org/10.1080/09546630600954594.
29. Gniadecki R, Kragballe K, Dam TN, Skov L. Comparison of drug survival rates for adalimumab, etanercept and infliximab in patients with psoriasis vulgaris. Br J Dermatol. 2011;164(5):1091–6. https://doi.org/10.1111/j.1365-2133.2011.10213.x.
30. Esposito M, Gisondi P, Cassano N, Ferrucci G, Del Giglio M, Loconsole F, et al. Survival rate of antitumour necrosis factor-α treatments for psoriasis in routine dermatological practice: a multicentre observational study. Br J Dermatol. 2013;169(3):666–72. https://doi.org/10.1111/bjd.12422.
31. Vide J, Magina S. Moderate to severe psoriasis treatment challenges through the era of biological drugs. An Bras Dermatol. 2017;92(5):668–74. https://doi.org/10.1590/abd1806-4841.20175603.
32. Kim WB, Marinas JEC, Qiang J, Shahbaz A, Greaves S, Yeung J. Adverse events resulting in withdrawal of biologic therapy for psoriasis in real-world clinical practice: a Canadian multicenter retrospective study. J Am Acad Dermatol. 2015;73(2):237–41. https://doi.org/10.1016/j.jaad.2015.04.023.
33. Armstrong AW, Robertson AD, Wu J, Schupp C, Lebwohl MG. Undertreatment, treatment trends, and treatment dissatisfaction among patients with psoriasis and psoriatic arthritis in the United States: findings from the National Psoriasis Foundation surveys, 2003-2011. JAMA Dermatol. 2013;149(10):1180–5. https://doi.org/10.1001/jamadermatol.2013.5264.
34. López-Ferrer A, Vilarrasa E, Gich IJ, Puig L. Adalimumab for the treatment of psoriasis in real life: a retrospective cohort of 119 patients at a single Spanish centre. Br J Dermatol. 2013;169(5):1141–7. https://doi.org/10.1111/bjd.12543.
35. Puig L, Ruiz-Salas V. Long-term efficacy, safety and drug survival of ustekinumab in a Spanish cohort of patients with moderate to severe plaque psoriasis. Dermatology. 2015;230(1):46–54. https://doi.org/10.1159/000366499.
36. Inzinger M, Wippel-Slupetzky K, Weger W, Richter L, Mlynek A, Fleischander B, et al. Survival and effectiveness of tumour necrosis factor-alpha inhibitors in the treatment of plaque psoriasis under daily life conditions: report from the Psoriasis Registry Austria. Acta Derm Venereol. 2016;96(2):207–12. https://doi.org/10.2340/00015555-2214.
37. Goren A, Carter C, Lee S. Patient reported health outcomes and non-adherence in psoriasis patients receiving adalimumab or ustekinumab for moderate to severe plaque psoriasis. J Dermatolog Treat. 2016;27(1):43–50. https://doi.org/10.3109/09546634.2015.1049972.
38. Spertino J, Lopez-Ferrer A, Vilarrasa E, Puig L. Long-term study of infliximab for psoriasis in daily practice: drug survival depends on combined treatment, obesity and infusion reactions. J Eur Acad Dermatol Venereol. 2014;28(11):1514–21. https://doi.org/10.1111/jdv.12331.
39. Mocanu M, Toader MP, Rezus E, Taranu T. Aspects concerning patient adherence to anti-TNFα therapy in psoriasis: a decade of clinical experience. Exp Ther Med. 2019;18(6):4987–92. https://doi.org/10.3892/etm.2019.8008.
40. Lin P-T, Wang S-H, Chi C-C. Drug survival of biologics in treating psoriasis: a meta-analysis of real-world evidence. Sci Rep. 2018;8(1):16068. https://doi.org/10.1038/s41598-018-34293-y.
41. Feldman SR, Zhang J, Martinez DJ, Lopez-Gonzalez L, Marchlewicz EH, Shrady G, et al. Real-world treatment patterns and healthcare costs of biologics and apremilast among patients with moderate-to-severe plaque psoriasis by metabolic condition status. J Dermatolog Treat. 2021;32(2):203–11. https://doi.org/10.1080/09546634.2019.1698699.
42. Wu B, Muser E, Teeple A, Pericone CD, Feldman SR. Treatment adherence and persistence of five commonly prescribed medications for moderate to severe psoriasis in a U.S. commercially insured population. J Dermatol Treat. 2019;1-8 https://doi.org/10.1080/09546634.2019.1687828.
43. Clemmensen A, Spon M, Skov L, Zachariae C, Gniadecki R. Responses to ustekinumab in the anti-TNF agent-naïve vs. anti-TNF agent-exposed patients with psoriasis vulgaris. J Eur Acad

Dermatol Venereol. 2011;25(9):1037–40. https://doi.org/10.1111/j.1468-3083.2010.03914.x.
44. Ross C, Marshman G, Grillo M, Stanford T. Biological therapies for psoriasis: adherence and outcome analysis from a clinical perspective. Australas J Dermatol. 2016;57(2):137–40. https://doi.org/10.1111/ajd.12294.
45. Sandoval LF, Huang KE, Feldman SR. Adherence to ustekinumab in psoriasis patients. J Drugs Dermatol. 2013;12(10):1090–2.
46. Brownstone ND, Hong J, Mosca M, Hadeler E, Liao W, Bhutani T, et al. Biologic treatments of psoriasis: an update for the clinician. Biologics. 2021;15:39–51. https://doi.org/10.2147/BTT.S252578.
47. Hsu DY, Gniadecki R. Patient adherence to biologic agents in psoriasis. Dermatology. 2016;232(3):326–33. https://doi.org/10.1159/000444581.
48. Dávila-Seijo P, Dauden E, Carretero G, Ferrandiz C, Vanaclocha F, Gómez-García FJ, et al. Survival of classic and biological systemic drugs in psoriasis: results of the BIOBADADERM registry and critical analysis. J Eur Acad Dermatol Venereol. 2016;30(11):1942–50. https://doi.org/10.1111/jdv.13682.
49. Arnold T, Schaarschmidt M-L, Herr R, Fischer JE, Goerdt S, Peitsch WK. Drug survival rates and reasons for drug discontinuation in psoriasis. JDDG. J Dtsch Dermatol Ges. 2016;14(11):1089–99. https://doi.org/10.1111/ddg.13152.
50. Noiles K, Vender R. Biologic survival. J Drugs Dermatol. 2009;8(4):329–33.
51. West C, Narahari S, O'Neill J, Davis S, Huynh M, Clark A, et al. Adherence to adalimumab in patients with moderate to severe psoriasis. Dermatol Online J. 2013;19(5):18182.
52. Menting SP, Sitaram AS, Bonnerjee-van der Stok HM, de Rie MA, Hooft L, Spuls PI. Drug survival is not significantly different between biologics in patients with psoriasis vulgaris: a single-centre database analysis. Br J Dermatol. 2014;171(4):875–83. https://doi.org/10.1111/bjd.13001.
53. Umezawa Y, Nobeyama Y, Hayashi M, Fukuchi O, Ito T, Saeki H, et al. Drug survival rates in patients with psoriasis after treatment with biologics. J Dermatol. 2013;40(12):1008–13. https://doi.org/10.1111/1346-8138.12353.
54. Egeberg A, Ottosen MB, Gniadecki R, Broesby-Olsen S, Dam TN, Bryld LE, et al. Safety, efficacy and drug survival of biologics and biosimilars for moderate-to-severe plaque psoriasis. Br J Dermatol. 2018;178(2):509–19. https://doi.org/10.1111/bjd.16102.
55. Kromer C, Schaarschmidt M-L, Schmieder A, Herr R, Goerdt S, Peitsch WK. Patient preferences for treatment of psoriasis with biologicals: a discrete choice experiment. PLoS One. 2015;10(6):e0129120. https://doi.org/10.1371/journal.pone.0129120.
56. Oussedik E, Foy CG, Masicampo EJ, Kammrath LK, Anderson RE, Feldman SR. Accountability: a missing construct in models of adherence behavior and in clinical practice. Patient Prefer Adherence. 2017;11:1285–94. https://doi.org/10.2147/PPA.S135895.
57. Gelfand JM, Wang S, Takeshita J, Robertson AD, Krueger GG, Callis Duffin K, et al. Using Hawthorne effects to improve adherence in clinical practice: lessons from clinical trials--reply. JAMA Dermatol. 2013;149(4):491. https://doi.org/10.1001/jamadermatol.2013.2846.
58. Feldman SR, Camacho FT, Krejci-Manwaring J, Carroll CL, Balkrishnan R. Adherence to topical therapy increases around the time of office visits. J Am Acad Dermatol. 2007;57(1):81–3. https://doi.org/10.1016/j.jaad.2007.04.005.
59. Cramer JA, Scheyer RD, Mattson RH. Compliance declines between clinic visits. Arch Intern Med. 1990;150(7):1509–10.
60. Balato N, Megna M, Di Costanzo L, Balato A, Ayala F. Educational and motivational support service: a pilot study for mobile-phone-based interventions in patients with psoriasis. Br J Dermatol. 2013;168(1):201–5. https://doi.org/10.1111/j.1365-2133.2012.11205.x.
61. Oussedik E, Cardwell LA, Patel NU, Onikoyi O, Feldman SR. An anchoring-based intervention to increase patient willingness to use injectable medication in psoriasis. JAMA Dermatol. 2017;153(9):932–4. https://doi.org/10.1001/jamadermatol.2017.1271.
62. Aleshaki JS, Cardwell LA, Muse ME, Feldman SR. Adherence and resource use among psoriasis patients treated with biologics. Expert Rev Pharmacoecon Outcomes Res. 2018;18(6):609–17. https://doi.org/10.1080/14737167.2018.1512408.
63. Lam WY, Fresco P. Medication adherence measures: an overview. Biomed Res Int. 2015;2015:217047. https://doi.org/10.1155/2015/217047.
64. Honda H, Umezawa Y, Kikuchi S, Yanaba K, Fukuchi O, Ito T, et al. Switching of biologics in psoriasis: reasons and results. J Dermatol. 2017;44(9):1015–9. https://doi.org/10.1111/1346-8138.13860.
65. Marinas JE, Kim WB, Shahbaz A, Qiang JK, Greaves S, Yeung J. Survival rates of biological therapies for psoriasis treatment in real-world clinical practice: a Canadian multicentre retrospective study. Australas J Dermatol. 2018;59(1):e11–e4. https://doi.org/10.1111/ajd.12548.
66. Belinchón I, Rivera R, Blanch C, Comellas M, Lizán L. Adherence, satisfaction and preferences for treatment in patients with psoriasis in the European Union: a systematic review of the literature. Patient Prefer Adherence. 2016;10:2357–67. https://doi.org/10.2147/PPA.S117006.
67. Lewis DJ, Cardwell LA, Feldman SR. Applying behavioural economics to psoriasis treatment: interventions to improve patient adherence to biologics. J Eur Acad Dermatol Venereol. 2018;32(2):e65–e6. https://doi.org/10.1111/jdv.14504.
68. Fenerty SD, West C, Davis SA, Kaplan SG, Feldman SR. The effect of reminder systems on patients' adherence to treatment. Patient Prefer Adherence. 2012;6:127–35. https://doi.org/10.2147/ppa.S26314.

Index

N. Brownstone et al. (eds.), *Biologic Therapy for Psoriasis*, Updates in Clinical Dermatology,
https://doi.org/10.1007/978-3-030-92938-1

GPSR Compliance

The European Union's (EU) General Product Safety Regulation (GPSR) is a set of rules that requires consumer products to be safe and our obligations to ensure this.

If you have any concerns about our products, you can contact us on ProductSafety@springernature.com

In case Publisher is established outside the EU, the EU authorized representative is:

Springer Nature Customer Service Center GmbH
Europaplatz 3
69115 Heidelberg, Germany

Batch number: 10731395

Printed by Printforce, the Netherlands